PREVENTION

PREVENTIONITIS

*The exaggerated claims of
health promotion*

Edited by
James Le Fanu

THE SOCIAL AFFAIRS UNIT

British Library Cataloguing in Publication Data
A cataloguing record of this book is available from
the British Library

ISBN 0 907631 58 4

Book production by Crowley Esmonde Ltd
Typeset by Rowland Phototypesetting Ltd, Bury St Edmunds, Suffolk
Printed and bound in Great Britain by
St Edmundsbury Press Ltd, Bury St Edmunds, Suffolk

Contents

The Authors   7

Preface   10
Digby Anderson

1 Introduction and summary   12
James Le Fanu

2 Prevention: wishful thinking or hard science?   23
James Le Fanu

**3 The need for caution in interpreting low level risks
reported by epidemiologists**   36
Peter Lee

**4 Health promotion and NHS reform: a critique of
*Health of the Nation***   46
Bruce Charlton

5 Prevention and clinical freedom: a clinician's view   56
John Hampton

**6 High blood cholesterol: a problem with no
ready solution**   64
L E Ramsay, W W Yeo and P R Jackson

**7 *Health of the Nation*: a critical appraisal of
Government policy on mental health**   81
Frank Holloway

8 Does health education work?   89
James Le Fanu

9 The costs of screening   106
Mark Charny

10 The ethics of prevention   118
Petr Skrabanek

Notes and References   128

The Authors

Dr Bruce Charlton MD is lecturer in public health medicine at the University of Newcastle-upon-Tyne. He has published numerous articles, essays and reviews on subjects such as psychiatry, philosophy, public health, epidemiology, English literature and education. He wrote an 'experimental' Radio 3 broadcast entitled *Solitude, exile and ecstasy*, and is co-author of *The Making of a Doctor* (with R S Downie).

Dr Mark Charny is Director of Public Health for the Wiltshire and Bath Health Commission. He has published extensively on the cost-effectiveness of services and on public views on a wide range of issues. He has taken a particular interest in screening. More recently he has been developing a health programme approach to decision-making in which an overview of *all* potential contributions to a health problem is taken. This allows prevention to take its proper place, but he believes that this place must be earned and not given by virtue of philosophical principle.

Professor John Hampton is currently Professor of Cardiology at Nottingham University, Clinical Director of Medicine at the Queen's Medical Centre and Consultant Physician to the Nottingham Hospitals. Having graduated from Oxford University he undertook his clinical training at the Radcliffe Infirmary. Before moving to Nottingham he held appointments at the Royal Postgraduate Medical School in Oxford and at Harvard University. His main research interests are clinical epidemiology and clinical trials in cardiovascular disease.

Dr Frank Holloway is Consultant Psychiatrist at the Maudsley Hospital in South London. He was formerly MRC Training Fellow in Social Psychiatry in the Academic Department of Physiological Medicine at King's College, London. He co-edited *Community Care in Practice, Services for the Continuing Care Client* (with A Lavender) and has contributed articles on government policy for the mentally ill to *Psychiatric Bulletin* and on case management to *The International Journal of Social Psychiatry*.

Dr P R Jackson is currently Senior Lecturer in Medicine and Pharmacology at the University of Sheffield and Honorary Consultant Physician at the Royal Hallamshire Hospital. He was previously MRC Fellow in Clinical Pharmacology. His interests include the interaction between mathematics and clinical pharmacology and medicine. Clinically he jointly runs a busy general medical unit, as well as the Sheffield Hypertension Clinic.

Dr James Le Fanu, a graduate of Cambridge University, is medical columnist of *The Sunday Telegraph*, a weekly contributor to *The Times* and the *Daily Telegraph*, and is a general practitioner in London. He is author of a number of books and reports, including *Eat Your Heart Out, Healthwise: An Intelligent Guide for the Over 60s* and *Environmental Alarums: A medical audit of environmental damage to human health*. He has also contributed numerous articles to edited books and journals.

Peter Lee studied mathematics and statistics at Oxford University, gaining his MA in 1969. He worked as a statistician and then research co-ordinator before becoming an independent consultant in statistics and adviser in epidemiology and toxicology and forming his own company, P N Lee Statistics and Computing Ltd, which carries out medical statistical work for a wide range of clients. He has published four books and well over 100 papers and letters. Effects of passive smoking are a particular research interest.

Professor Lawrence Ramsay is Professor of Clinical Pharmacology and Therapeutics at the University of Sheffield and Consultant Physician in the Royal Hallamshire Hospital. He is jointly Director of the Sheffield Hypertension Clinic and has a clinical and research interest in hypertension and prevention of cardiovascular disease. He has published numerous papers on these and other topics. He is Editor of the *British Journal of Clinical Pharmacology* and lately was Secretary of the British Hypertension Society.

Professor Petr Skrabanek is a Fellow of Trinity College Dublin and a Fellow of the Royal College of Physicians in Ireland. He is author of over 300 publications. His latest book, *Follies and Fallacies in Medicine*, has been translated into Danish, Dutch, French, German, Italian and Spanish.

Dr W W Yeo is currently Lecturer in Medicine and Clinical Pharmacology at the University of Sheffield and honorary Senior Registrar in Medicine at the Royal Hallamshire Hospital. His clinical and research interests include the evaluation of therapeutic strategies to prevent ischaemic heart disease and stroke, and the clinical assessment of new and established cardiovascular drugs. His other interests include programmes which aim to develop undergraduate and postgraduate medical education, particularly those concerned with applying the results of major therapeutic trials to optimise patient care.

Preface

Preventionitis seeks to assess the worth of the preventive policies of *Health of the Nation*. The general verdict is that while some preventive medicine works, much does not. Moreover, the costs of its failures are high, challenging the dogma that prevention is cheaper than cure.

The possibilities of prevention are limited by the fact that most of us 'live out our natural lifespan to die of diseases powerfully determined by ageing . . . The gains that can be made are small . . . The rise in life expectancy for those between the ages of 15 and 65 from preventing or curing all cancers – even if this were possible – would be only seven months.' Preventive policies are further limited by their chief knowledge base, epidemiology, which is prolific in raising possible associations between disease and lifestyle factors but poor in proving many of them. There is, for instance, strong evidence about the dangers of smoking but much weaker evidence about passive smoking or about the links between diet and heart disease. Even where strong links are established, they offer little guide to what can be done. Much health education is ineffective and particular screening programmes for breast and cervical cancer are of dubious efficacy.

One author argues that the policies are too weak and that more coercion and economic direction are needed to make people change to a 'healthier' way of life. Others point out that the preventive policies are dirigiste and sit uneasily with the Government's other policies of individual choice and liberty.

It seems the current prevention strategy manages to be both intrusive and ineffective.

It also raises ethical worries. Unlike curative medicine, health promotion is not restrained by a code of ethics. Many people are needlessly worried by certain screening programmes and unproven claims about health hazards. One chapter proposes that health promotionists should have to attach their own health warnings pointing out that 'the effectiveness of this advice has not been confirmed by medical trials' and that patients not informed of the *cons* as well as the pros of screening programmes should have the right to sue for 'dignitary tort'.

The governments of advanced countries are investing heavily in health promotion as part of a public health strategy. It is not the old, well-founded public health that has a proven record in dramatically reducing disease, the public health that relied on hard science and engineering, as in the provision of clean water. It is a new prevention which relies on social science, mass persuasion and the manipulation of people. The opinion of these authors suggests that governments ought to evaluate health promotion's worth, its failures, costs and, indeed, dangers very much more carefully before diverting resources from tried and tested curative medicine.

The views expressed by individual authors are their own, not those of the Social Affairs Unit, its Director or Trustees. Nevertheless I warmly commend them as a spur to much needed public debate.

Digby Anderson 1994

Introduction and Summary

James Le Fanu

Distinguishing effective from ineffective prevention
'For every problem there is a solution – neat, plausible and wrong' the American, H L Mencken famously observed. With medicine the 'problem' is clear – escalating demands for health care from an increasingly elderly and demanding population, escalating possibilities for meeting those needs in the form of improved drugs, operations and imaging techniques, but a limit, now universally acknowledged, to the resources that can be put towards them.

The 'solution' – greater emphasis on 'preventing disease rather than curing it' – is both neat and plausible. Prevention is, after all, widely believed to be 'cheaper' and 'better' – 'a penny of prevention is worth a pound spent on cure'. But, *pace* Mr Mencken, is the solution right or wrong?

The answer is probably both 'yes' and 'no' and it is important to distinguish valid claims for the preventability of disease from those which are not. This has become a matter of some urgency because over the last decade those in a position to influence health policy have come to believe very strongly in the virtues of prevention and have, through the White Paper, *Health of the Nation*, mobilised both energy and resources to implementing appropriate policies. Where this commitment to prevention is soundly based it is highly commendable but where it is not, the consequences can be serious both in distorting the priorities of the health service and in squandering resources that would be better spent elsewhere. It is certainly necessary to take a critical look at current prevention policies – something which, perhaps surprisingly, has not previously been attempted. It is this omission that the contributors to this collection set out to redress.

Only limited health gains possible

The possibilities and opportunities to influence patterns of disease are seriously constrained by the fact that for the first time in human history most people in our society live out their natural lifespan to die from diseases powerfully determined by ageing – cancers and diseases of the circulatory system, such as stroke and coronary heart disease. So the gains that can be made by such desirable goals as the elimination of cancer must be fairly small. Indeed, it has been calculated that the rise in life expectancy for those between the ages of 15 and 65 from preventing or curing all cancers – even if this were possible – would be only seven months.

This does not mean that within this major group of diseases there might not be some in which the evidence of specific causation is so overwhelming that prevention might be relatively straightforward, but clearly we have to look closely at the evidence to ascertain which these are.

The quality of the scientific evidence on which the claims for prevention of disease are based is the concern of the first two chapters. Dr Le Fanu points out that claims that, for example, smoking causes lung cancer (and therefore encouraging people to stop smoking might prevent the disease) are based on the 'canons' of epidemiological proof set out by the late Sir Austin Bradford Hill. These canons seek to assess the quality and internal consistency of any association between some aspect of the environment and disease. Assessing the evidence of the correlation between smoking and lung cancer in the light of Sir Austin's canons it is found to be plausible, strong, consistent, to contain a biological dose-response relationship, to hold over time and to have been confirmed by experiment insofar as those who stop smoking predictably reduce their subsequent risk of developing the disease.

Inadequate evidence and too many risks
However, when the gold standard of these canons is used to examine correlations between other risk factors and their associated diseases, such as the role of diet in cancer, fat consumption in heart disease, or salt in raised blood pressure, the evidence is either lacking or fails to demonstrate the required qualities of coherence and internal consistency.

This failure, Dr Le Fanu argues, presents a fundamental and frequently overlooked problem – the desire that any particular disease might be, or indeed should be, prevented is no substitute for the absolute requirement that the scientific evidence of specific causality be clear and unambiguous.

This theme is further developed by Peter Lee who assesses the epidemiological evidence surrounding the so-called 'risks of everyday life' in which a bewildering array of diseases have been 'associated' with social factors: alcohol has been implicated in breast cancer; coffee in pancreatic cancer; aluminium in dementia; keeping cats in multiple sclerosis; the list is endless. Such alleged associations clearly imply that avoiding or mitigating these hazards might in some way prevent the diseases developing.

Taking the example of the alleged link between passive smoking and lung cancer, Lee describes the many ways in which 'incautious and possibly incorrect claims have been made due to a failure to take into account the limitations of epidemiology'. How vigorously, for example, have other potential explanations for the findings ('confounders') been excluded. 'In a recent study', he writes, 'comparing heavy smokers with lifelong non-smokers in respect of the presence of 33 factors commonly associated with an adverse effect on health, it was observed that the heavy smokers were significantly worse off in respect of no less than 27 of these (*inter alia*, they were less educated, of lower social class, worked more often in occupations with a cancer risk . . .) . . . living with a smoker was clearly associated with many of these adverse factors . . . [which] were capable, if not taken into account, of distorting the relationship of both smoking and passive smoking with a range of diseases'.

In interpreting the results of any study, Lee concludes, 'epidemiologists should also be much more aware that an association between a disease and an agent can only be regarded as evidence of a cause-and-effect relationship if *all* alternative explanations can be ruled out'.

The politics of prevention versus the politics of NHS reform
There is an inescapable political element in the present Government's commitment to preventive policies as laid out in *Health of the Nation*. The validity of the belief that 'prevention' is an alternative to and should be given higher priority as a cheaper and better way of improving the nation's health than practical clinical medicine is examined by Dr Bruce Charlton and Professor John Hampton.

First, Dr Charlton, lecturer in Public Health at the University of Newcastle-upon-Tyne, points out that there is in fact a fundamental and irreconcilable ideological conflict between the two major prongs of Government health policy. The perspective in *Health of the Nation* is of a planned health service in which targets are set at the top, its resemblance to 'the "rationalistic" world of classical "scientific socialism" is too obvious to escape comment', claims Dr Charlton, and its emphasis on central planning 'is reminiscent of the simple certainties of a bygone era'.

Further, many of the principles underlying preventive strategies are inimicable to the values of a free society. They are 'dirigiste', intrude on a citizen's life and liberties by upbraiding and cajoling him to switch from an allegedly 'unhealthy' to an allegedly 'healthier' lifestyle. Whether this is a legitimate arena of state interest is a question which is rarely, if ever, posed. And this socialist, or at least liberal philosophy is even more remarkable when compared with the 1990 NHS reforms which drew their inspiration from the opposite end of the political spectrum where it is believed that the creation of an internal market in health will, by encouraging competition, improve the quality of the services provided by the NHS. According to Dr Charlton 'both strategies are utopian, reductionist and ideological – based on ideas of what "ought" to work, rather than developing from what actually does work'. He argues that a more sensible approach would be based on the traditional conservative principles of preserving 'the benefits of past practice while trying to discard only the deficiencies'.

Politics – as the language of priorities – is also the theme of Professor Hampton's contribution. 'Once we do start talking about choices', he says, 'we can see straight away that a choice will have to be made between prevention and treatment. Prevention is not simply a cheaper alternative . . . Preventing a case of most diseases costs as much or more than treating the effects of that disease in an individual'.

So how are these choices to be made? Professor Hampton argues that exactly the same criteria that are applied to assessing the efficacy of clinical practice – particularly the evidence from clinical trials – should be applied to preventive measures. Preventive medicine is 'just another form of "treatment", different only in that it is healthy subjects that are being "treated" and not patients with established disease; prevention is just another choice'.

The practicalities of prevention, particularly whether recommendations for a shift to a 'healthy' diet can, by lowering cholesterol levels, reduce the risk of heart disease and whether the goals of a reduction in suicide can be achieved by preventive means, are examined by Professor Ramsay and his colleagues and by Dr Frank Holloway.

Cholesterol guidance not supported by evidence

Professor Ramsay and Drs Jackson and Yeo from the University of Sheffield's Department of Medicine and Pharmacology have long been interested in the possibilities of preventing strokes by identifying and treating those subjects with raised blood pressure. 'After 30 years' they can report, 'we have a fair idea of the strengths and limitations of treatment . . . Remarkably during that time "current wisdom" was often – even usually – proved wrong by the results of . . . controlled [clinical] trials'.

As many patients with raised blood pressure also had raised cholesterol levels, the authors were forced to take an interest in the claims that cholesterol levels could be reduced by changes in diet. But 'to our astonishment', they write, 'the average reduction of blood cholesterol was not the 10–25 per cent suggested – it was in fact a cholesterol fall of only two per cent . . . In only one of these trials was the fall in blood cholesterol statistically significant. A fall in blood cholesterol of this magnitude would have a negligible impact on coronary risk'. Their conclusion is that guidelines for managing high cholesterol levels are not supported by the scientific evidence and are seriously flawed. Put simply, 'there is no form of treatment to lower high blood cholesterol which is effective, feasible, acceptable and safe'.

Dr Frank Holloway of the Maudsley Hospital takes issue with the belief that suicide is readily preventable. Rather, he claims, 'there is . . . absolutely no evidence that the onset of serious mental illness can be prevented'.

He draws attention to what he sees as the fundamental problem in providing services for the mentally ill that are 'comprehensive, local and integrated'. He points out that, paradoxically, such provision has been made considerably more, not less difficult to achieve by the other, contradictory, arm of Government health strategy – the internal market with its emphasis on encouraging competition between 'purchasers and providers', 'health and social services', 'the hospital and the community'. As a result, he says, 'it is possible that current trends in psychiatric practice may actually increase the risk of suicide amongst patients in contact with services'.

The main criticism of the current enthusiasm for prevention is the dissonance between the laudable aims of its protagonists and the hard evidence that such aims are achieveable. This is particularly the case with the two principle mechanisms of preventive strategies – health education and screening.

Ineffective health education: heart disease and AIDS

Health education is, as Dr Le Fanu points out, 'qualitatively different from most other forms of education whose aim is to impart knowledge or intellectual skills. It is not enough simply to educate the public about, say, the dangers of saturated fat, health education has to go further and actually get people to act on that knowledge. This . . . is unlikely to be easy'. The main mechanism for achieving many of the desirable goals of disease prevention rests on the assumption that health education can achieve changes in people's lives which leads to an apparently paradoxical, but very important observation. Studies of the effectiveness of health education show that on the whole it does not work very well yet certain quite dramatic changes in the pattern of disease, notably the decline in coronary heart disease and containing the AIDS epidemic have been attributed to it. It is therefore necessary to examine in some detail the statistics of these diseases with which such spectacular success has been claimed.

Coronary heart disease, for example, has declined by almost 50 per cent in the United States, Canada and Australia and a similar pattern is now being observed in several countries in Western Europe. For this to be attributed to the ability of health education to encourage people to shift to a 'healthier lifestyle' and, in particular, a healthy diet, it would be necessary to demonstrate a parallel change in the pattern of food consumption. But this is not possible. Massive changes both in the rise and subsequent fall of coronary heart disease over the last 50 years have only been accompanied by a trivial change in fat consumption as a percentage of energy intake. The only logical interpretation therefore, is that the correlation between changing patterns of heart disease and dietary change is an example of the *post hoc – ergo propter hoc* fallacy where, because the decline appears to coincide with 'trends' towards a healthy lifestyle, so the disease itself is attributed to an 'unhealthy' lifestyle.

The case of AIDS is quite different because there have quite clearly been marked changes in the patterns of 'unsafe' sexual practices, especially amongst male homosexuals, as measured by 'markers' of the disease such as the incidence of rectal gonorrhoea. However, it seems indisputable that the major shift towards safe sex occurred well before the first high-profile health education campaigns directed at preventing AIDS. Therefore the 'containment' of the epidemic cannot justifiably be attributed to those campaigns. 'The answer to the question "does health education work"', concludes Dr Le Fanu, 'is, regrettably, very rarely'.

Limited uses of screening
The arguments in favour of screening to diagnose diseases such as breast and cervical cancer in the hope that sufficiently early detection will render them more readily treatable or, indeed, curable, are both plausible and sensible. Dr Mark Charny, Director of Public Health for the Wiltshire and Bath Health Commission takes a bold march through the uncertain assumptions, daunting organisational problems and heavy financial costs of screening programmes. He questions whether the aims of such programmes are achievable, either theoretically or logistically, or whether their complexity is such as to prevent their having any substantial effect.

Screening certainly can work. Two programmes in particular prove this – testing for congenital hypothyroidism in the prevention of cretinism, and testing for phenylketonuria thus preventing the mental backwardness associated with that condition. Both these examples, however, fully comply with the well-established principles – ten in all – that need to be fulfilled for a screening programme to be effective. There has to be a suitable and acceptable test; the natural history of the disease must be adequately understood; an intervention of proven value must exist; and so on.

However, problems arise when other important screening programmes, notably for breast and cervical cancer and for raised cholesterol in the blood are examined in the light of these principles. The interpretation of the cervical smear for example, as Dr Charny points out, is not straightforward. Research has repeatedly shown that pathologists reading the same set of smears not only frequently disagree with each other, but even with themselves!

The problem with screening for breast cancer is that by the time the tumour reaches a size detectable by mammography 'it has been estimated . . . that it may have been present for an average of nine years'. It is therefore necessary to assume that, if breast screening is to be effective, the lethal metastatic spread of the tumour does not occur during this time and though this is possible, it is, says Dr Charny, 'intrinsically unlikely'.

He argues that cholesterol screening is limited in its effectiveness because 'there is no agreement among experts as to whether an effective treatment exists for those with moderately raised blood cholesterol levels'. He concludes, 'By being more critical we can promote those [screening programmes] that really work and avoid the harm caused by those that do not work, including the harm that wasted resources do to others who need services which cannot be funded as a result'.

No ethical controls on prevention
Finally, Professor Petr Skrabanek of Trinity College, Dublin examines the ethics of prevention. He looks at the anomaly by which preventive measures are exempted from the guidelines governing consent to treatment or participation in medical experiments because of the 'widely accepted notion that if it is "prevention" it must be good, and therefore the usual ethical constraints do not apply'. Prevention is, however, not intrinsically 'a good thing' and in different ways has breached the four pillars on which medical ethics are founded – 'non-maleficence, beneficence, autonomy and justice'.

Professor Skrabanek observes that 'It is not widely appreciated that "preventive" measures can prove disastrous'. These include the swine-flu vaccination programme in the United States which resulted in serious neurological complications in more than 500 people, and increased mortality rates in patients given drugs either to control heart disease or high cholesterol levels.

A further ethical problem associated with prevention is the tendency to label normal physiological parameters such as weight, blood pressure and alcohol consumption as 'abnormal', with the result that everybody becomes a patient and has to change their lifestyle according to the preventionists' diktat. Professor Skrabanek suggests that, in line with other forms of medical intervention, the formal consent of potential participants in prevention programmes should first be sought. Further, mass media campaigns should be obliged to reflect the scientific claims on which they are based. For example, campaigns promoting a healthy diet as a means of preventing coronary heart disease would have to point out that 'the effectiveness of this advice has not been confirmed by medical trials'. Doctors who fail to inform patients of the pros and cons of screening programmes for breast or cervical cancer should be liable to 'dignitary tort', as in the United States, for affronting the patients' dignity by preventing them from

21

exercising their rights to rational participation. Further, protection of the participant in any preventive measures should be provided by a written form, signed by the doctor and describing the accuracy of the test, the probability of benefit and the probability and nature of adverse outcomes. Finally, Dr Skrabanek urges that a forum be set up 'at which representatives of the public and of the medical and legal professions would identify the ethical problems of prevention and draw up guidelines for protecting the public against unethical practices'.

Prevention: wishful thinking or hard science?

James Le Fanu

Real limits on preventive medicine

There is a beguiling complementarity in the two great projects of modern medicine – the prevention and treatment of disease. The methods and achievements of prevention have recently been elegantly and convincingly demonstrated in the commonest cause of post-neonatal mortality – sudden infant death syndrome (SIDS). This condition, by definition, cannot be treated and so the only way its incidence could be reduced was by prevention, which in turn requires an understanding of its cause. Diligent research in the last ten years has pointed to a host of potential candidates. Was it caused by a virus infection? Or some subtle abnormality of the respiratory centre in the brain? Or fungal spores in the mattresses on which babies slept? Then a chance observation that SIDS had markedly increased following a change in advice to parents that babies should sleep prone rather than supine raised the possibility that sleeping position might be crucial. And so it turned out. A highly publicised campaign encouraging parents to place their babies on their backs was followed almost immediately by a precipitous 40 per cent decline in SIDS.[1]

This, of course, is only the latest in a long and impressive list of the achievements of preventive medicine that stretch from the great sanitary reforms of the last century to the elimination by vaccination of the life-threatening infectious diseases of childhood – tetanus, polio and diphtheria.

On the other hand, and self evidently, a completely different intellectual approach, mostly empirical and technical, has resulted in the revolutionary transformation of the treatment of disease since the Second World War. A cornucopia of new drugs and operations considerably alleviate the problems associated with the chronic degenerative diseases of ageing – heart disease, arthritis, cataracts – which are not amenable to prevention but are rather a necessary result of the marked general increase in life expectancy.

In an ideal world there would be both preventive and therapeutic medicine. But the world is not ideal. An ageing population and new and often costly therapeutic discoveries have placed demands on clinical services that cannot be fully met with current resources, thus leading to a need to ration them by waiting lists or, more drastically, by administrative decisions about what sort of drugs and operations should be permitted and for whom. This in turn has given rise to an idea that has proved very seductive to politicians, that prevention and treatment are not complementary, rather prevention is better and cheaper. Put another way, substantial resources that go on treatment would be better directed towards prevention.

Prevention in some cases, for example lung cancer or AIDS, can certainly be dramatically better and cheaper than 'cure'. Preventive measures that encourage safe sex or giving up smoking are, if they work, cheaper by several orders of magnitude. The contrast between the effectiveness of prevention and the relative ineffectiveness of white-coated doctors with their potent remedies, no matter how hard-working and assiduous they may be, further fuels the conviction that 'prevention' is superior.

In *Health of the Nation*, published in 1992, this belief in the virtues of prevention is clearly evident in the policy of setting targets – the rate of stroke and coronary heart disease is set to fall by 40 per cent by the year 2000; the problem of obesity in men by 25 per cent; the number of suicides to decline by a third; conceptions in those under 16 by a half; and so on.[2] This, however, is deceptive. There is a sense that by sleight of hand a serious problem – for example, how we are to find the resources to cut the waiting list for open heart surgery – is transformed into a 'non-problem'. If prevention can reduce heart disease by 40 per cent, then the demands for the services of cardio-thoracic surgeons will be reduced.

There then arises a conflict of interest between the priorities of the health service, as perceived by those controlling health policy, and the ordinary man in the street. The public are not interested in 'prevention goals' but think rather that the National Health Service should look after them when they are ill. But these every day needs for care, surgery and medicines are not prioritised, targeted or focused on in the same way as the goals for prevention set out in Government policy. Rather public access to them are to be left to the vagaries of the 'internal market' in health. From the public's perspective therefore, whether or not they are aware of it, it becomes a matter of some importance to know whether the preventionist strategies laid out in *Health of the Nation* are intellectually coherent. Is prevention really better than or an alternative to cure? What are the 'limits of prevention', and how can one tell?

Clearly the opportunities for a preventive approach to influencing patterns of disease are seriously constrained by the fact that we live in a society where, for the first time in recorded history, most people live out their natural life-span to die from diseases powerfully determined by ageing – notably cancer and diseases of the circulatory system. So the gains that can be achieved by such desirable goals as the elimination of cancer or the prevention of heart disease are fairly small. It has been calculated that the gain in average life-span for those between the ages of 15 and 65 from preventing all cancers (were this possible) would be seven months.[3] In Sweden, for example, the median age of death for men from cancer is 74 and from other causes is 76; for women the median age of death from cancer is 75 and from all other causes it is over 80. The median age for death from coronary heart disease for men is 74 and for women 82.[4]

Prevention requires knowledge of the causes of diseases
This does not mean that within this major group of diseases, there might not be some in which the evidence of specific causation is so overwhelming that prevention should be relatively straightforward. Nor does it mean that it might not be possible to postpone death from these diseases by appropriate preventive measures. Nor indeed that there are not other important categories of illness, notably the sexually-transmitted diseases and accidents, that are amenable to preventive measures. This however should not obscure the fundamental fact that the overall benefit from prevention is likely to be small or, put another way, that it cannot replace or supplant the pressing requirement on the health service to continue treating the illnesses that afflict people.

The next question that arises then, is how do we distinguish the specific types of circulatory disorder or cancer that might be amenable to a preventive strategy. The answer is quite clear: by knowing their cause. If the specific cause of a cancer is known, it can usually be prevented. If it is not known, it cannot. Now the specific cause of one type of cancer – lung cancer – is known. The evidence of its association with smoking is not only very strong – a twentyfold increased risk – it is also highly internally consistent, that is, in whatever way one looks at the relationship, it is still very marked. To be precise, the smoking/lung cancer link fulfills the 'canons of epidemiological proof' as laid down by the late Sir Austin Bradford Hill, and which are based on elementary rules of logic.[5]

This is crucial because in the enthusiasm for preventing disease a whole series of 'associations' have been found;[6] so many indeed that they have been caricatured as being the 'menaces of everyday life'. Coffee is linked with cancer of the pancreas; alcohol with breast cancer; grilled steak with stomach cancer; and, of course, fat with heart disease. There has to be some way of distinguishing those associations that are truly causal from those that are just 'associations'.

The proofs prevention needs

By examining the smoking/lung cancer 'association' in terms of Bradford Hill's canons of epidemiological proof we get a gold standard against which other 'associations' can be measured, thus giving an idea of whether they are preventable or not.

The correlation is biologically plausible: there are cancer-inducing agents in tobacco that, when brought in contact with lung tissue, could cause the disease.

The correlation is strong: the death rate from lung cancer in cigarette smokers is 20 times that in non-smokers.

The correlation reflects a biological gradient: the more cigarettes that are smoked, the higher the risk of lung cancer.

The correlation is found consistently: 36 separate studies examining the relationship between smoking and lung cancer have found a positive correlation.

The correlation has held over time: as cigarette consumption has steadily increased it has been parallelled by a rise in incidence of the disease.

The association is confirmed by experiment: according to Bradford Hill, 'here the strongest support for a causative hypothesis will be found'. As smoking causes lung cancer, stopping smoking reduces that risk; and the longer the time elapses since stopping smoking, the lower that risk.

So we have progressed from a well-recognised association, that people who smoke get lung cancer, to a scientific certainty, that smoking causes lung cancer. Bradford Hill's canons would only have been fulfilled were that the case. There might of course be additional causes for the disease. A rare type of lung cancer can occur in non-smokers. The disease is commoner in urban than rural areas so perhaps pollution plays a role. Not everyone who smokes develops the disease, so perhaps certain people are protected in some way by their genes. But these observations are insufficient to annul the massive, overpowering statistical evidence that smoking causes the disease. Bradford Hill's canons are similarly fulfilled for asbestosis and lung cancer, and air pollution and bronchitis, but when the same gold standard is applied to other allegedly preventable causes of disease, they are not.

So what about another central tenet of preventive strategies, that a high fat diet causes heart disease. How does this thesis fare when the rigours of Bradford Hill's canons are applied? Certainly the first criteria seems valid enough. It is biologically plausible that fat in the diet might, by raising cholesterol levels in the blood, accelerate narrowing of the arteries by atheroma and therefore cause heart disease. But beyond that the thesis does not fare so well. It should be possible to show that those who get heart disease eat more meat and dairy products than those who do not, and that the more of these fats consumed the greater the risk. This is not the case. The association should be found consistently, but it is not. Within Britain, for example, the Scots with a much higher incidence of heart disease actually consume less saturated fats than inhabitants of the South of England. There should be a correlation over time so the rise in heart disease in parts of the western hemisphere this century should be reflected in increasing dairy food and meat consumption, and its decline in the United States should be reflected by a decrease in the consumption of these foods. In fact, the rise and fall of heart disease over the last 50 years has been accompanied by only trivial changes in fat consumption. Finally, the thesis has been tested by experiment in massive 'risk factor intervention' trials but these have failed to reduce the risk of heart disease in those encouraged to lower the amount of fat in their diet.

The failure of the diet/heart thesis to fulfil Bradford Hill's canons presents a fundamental and frequently overlooked problem – that the hope that any particular disease might be, or indeed should be, prevented, cannot substitute for the absolute requirement that the scientific evidence of its causality must be clear and unambiguous. If it is not, then the preventive strategy will not work.

This then is the first 'limit of prevention'. The causes of death in our society are overwhelmingly age-determined and therefore not readily amenable to prevention. The identification of those that are preventable requires that the evidence of association with some aspect of environmental hazard or lifestyle is so overwhelming and so internally coherent that it can be truly categorised as causative.

When screening does not work
The second major method of prevention is by 'screening', that is, detecting diseases early enough for them to be more readily treatable or even curable. Once again it is necessary to emphasise the importance of scientific rigour. 'Screening' is the medical term, perhaps 'searching' is more appropriate. The doctor confronted by someone who is apparently outwardly healthy is searching for disease. In perhaps 95 per cent he will find nothing, and in another four per cent nothing of much consequence. In the remaining one per cent screening might detect raised blood pressure which if treated can prevent a stroke, or urine testing may show up asymptomatic diabetes. Further special tests like mammography or cervical screening can pick up cancers of the breast and cervix respectively, early enough for a cure to be possible.

PREVENTIONITIS

There is currently great enthusiasm for screening. The Government has recently written into the General Practitioners' Contract a requirement to screen the over 75s every three years and to offer all those joining their practice a simple health screen. The national breast and cervical screening programmes in which women are invited for tests on a regular basis are also vigorously promoted.

The enthusiasm for screening is commendable, but if resources are not to be wasted – and the screening programmes in particular can be very expensive – then it has to be assessed in a rigorous way by asking the obvious question: does it work? The answer is, needless to say, that it works for some illnesses but not others and for different reasons. Screening as a generalised principle as a means of preventing disease does not pass muster, it has to be taken item by item. Thus detecting very raised blood pressure and treating it with drugs has a dramatic and almost instantaneous effect in reducing death from stroke,[7] but the same is certainly not true for those with markedly raised cholesterol levels.[8] Screening by a simple blood test for hypothyroidism or phenylketonuria at birth is both cheap and prevents virtually 100 per cent of cases. By contrast, while there is some evidence from trials and in areas where the leadership of the programme is highly motivated, that screening for cervical and breast cancer may work, the complexity of the screening procedure, and the failure of those most likely to benefit to come forward to have the tests, means that, in Britain at least, the impact on these diseases is likely to be highly marginal.

This then is the second 'limit of prevention': though it is theoretically possible to prevent disease by screening, the complex logistics of screening programmes mean that the goal may not be achieved. (This will be referred to in greater detail in chapter 9.)

Finally, though preventing a disease may indeed be possible, we have to examine the means by which it can be achieved. Sanitary legislation has certainly eradicated major water-transmissible infectious diseases, but to control AIDS health education is necessary to encourage people to change their sexual habits. Similarly, smoking causes lung cancer but health education is necessary to persuade people to stop smoking. The scientifically rigorous question to be tackled here is, again, does it work? And again, as will be seen in chapter 8, the simple answer is, not very well.

When he was visiting a depressed area of South Wales between the Wars, the then Prince of Wales was told that tuberculosis was preventable, to which he perspicaciously responded, 'if preventable, why not prevented'. The answer was, of course, that TB was not truly preventable without two factors – a substantial increase in the standard of living, reduction of overcrowding and so on, and the discovery of anti-tuberculosis drugs which, when given to those infected, prevented its spread to others. In the post-War years both these criteria were fulfilled and TB became indeed 'preventable'.

We are faced with a similar question today in relation to the health of the nation and the Government's love affair with prevention. The diseases that are preventable are for the most part prevented and we should not for a moment forget the massive contribution that prevention has made to the high level of health we enjoy. This applies equally to the water-transmissible infections (prevented by legislation), the potentially lethal infective diseases of childhood (prevented by vaccination) and to hypothyroidism and phenylketonuria (prevented by screening).

If, however we turn to the list of prevention targets in the Government White Paper, *Health of the Nation*, the question as to why they are not prevented necessarily raises the issue of whether they are, in fact, preventable. And this can only be resolved by scrutinising the scientific evidence behind the targets. The targets are listed in *Table 1* and the means by which they are to be achieved – reduction of risk factors – in *Table 2*.

PREVENTIONITIS

Table 1: Health of the Nation main targets

Coronary heart disease and stroke*

To reduce death rates for both CHD and stroke in people under 65 by at least 40% by the year 2000 (*Baseline 1990*)

To reduce the death rate for CHD in people aged 65–74 by at least 30% by the year 2000 (*Baseline 1990*)

To reduce the death rate for stroke in people aged 65–74 by at least 40% by the year 2000 (*Baseline 1990*)

Cancers*

To reduce the death rate for breast cancer in the population invited for screening by at least 25% by the year 2000 (*Baseline 1990*)

To reduce the incidence of invasive cervical cancer by at least 20% by the year 2000 (*Baseline 1990*)

To reduce the death rate for lung cancer under the age of 75 by at least 30% in men and by at least 15% in women by 2010 (*Baseline 1990*)

To halt the year-on-year increase in the incidence of skin cancer by 2005

Mental illness*

To improve significantly the health and social functioning of mentally ill people

To reduce the overall suicide rate by at least 15% by the year 2000 (*Baseline 1990*)

To reduce the suicide rate of severely mentally ill people by at least 30% by the year 2000 (*Baseline 1990*)

HIV/AIDS and sexual health

To reduce the incidence of gonorrhoea by at least 20% by 1995 (*Baseline 1990*), as an indicator of HIV/AIDS trends

To reduce by at least 50% the rate of conceptions amongst the under 16s by the year 2000 (*Baseline 1989*)

Accidents*

To reduce the death rate for accidents among children aged under 15 by at least 33% by 2005 (*Baseline 1990*)

To reduce the death rate for accidents among young people aged 15–24 by at least 25% by 2005 (*Baseline 1990*)

To reduce the death rate for accidents among people aged 65 and over by at least 33% by 2005 (*Baseline 1990*)

* The 1990 baseline for all mortality targets represents an average of the three years centred around 1990.

Source: Department of Health, Health of the Nation, *HMSO, 1992*

Table 2: Health of the Nation risk factor targets

Smoking

To reduce the prevalence of cigarette smoking to no more than 20% by the year 2000 in both men and women (a reduction of a third) (*Baseline 1990*)

To reduce consumption of cigarettes by at least 40% by the year 2000 (*Baseline 1990*)

In addition to the overall reduction in prevalence, at least 33% of women smokers to stop smoking at the start of their pregnancy by the year 2000

To reduce smoking prevalence of 11–15 year-olds by at least 33% by 1994 (to less than 6%) (*Baseline 1988*)

Diet and Nutrition

To reduce the average percentage of food energy derived by the population from saturated fatty acids by at least 35% by 2005 (to no more than 11% of food energy) (*Baseline 1990*)

To reduce the average percentage of food energy derived from total fat by the population by at least 12% by 2005 (to no more than about 35% of total food energy) (*Baseline 1990*)

To reduce the proportion of men and women aged 16–64 who are obese by at least 25% and 33% respectively by 2005 (to no more than 6% of men and 8% of women) (*Baseline 1986/87*)

To reduce the proportion of men drinking more than 21 units of alcohol per week and women drinking more than 14 units per week by 30% by 2005 (to 18% of men and 7% of women) (*Baseline 1990*)

Blood Pressure

To reduce mean systolic blood pressure in the adult population by at least 5mm Hg by 2005 (*Baseline to be derived from new national health survey*)

HIV/AIDS

To reduce the percentage of injecting drug misusers who report sharing injecting equipment in the previous 4 weeks from 20% in 1990 to no more than 10% by 1997 and no more than 5% by the year 2000

Source: Department of Health, Health of the Nation, *HMSO, 1992*

Both the targets and the means by which they are to be achieved appear to fall into three broad categories.

Category one: potentially achievable

- *Smoking and lung cancer:* reduction of smoking as outlined would definitely result in a fall in lung cancer, the only question is the degree to which health education can promote this goal. After all, nobody needs to be 'educated' about the harm of smoking, everyone knows. The huge social stigmatisation of smokers, especially in the promotion of the potential harm of 'passive smoking' is likely to be more effective.

- *Raised blood pressure and strokes:* the fall in death rate from stroke is achievable by the systematic identification and treatment of those with raised blood pressure. Interestingly, the means of achieving this goal is not mentioned, instead the 'mean blood pressure' in the adult population has to fall by at least '5mms of mercury'. It is not clear how this is to be done, nor indeed whether 'mean falls' of any physiological parameter are achievable and, if they were, whether they would have any effect on strokes.

- *Screening for cervical and breast cancer:* the targets outlined here are remarkably modest, especially those for cervical cancer, and presumably reflect the awareness that expensive as these screening programmes might be, the logistical problems in carrying them out means that they are much less effective than is desirable.

Category two: potentially achievable but mechanism not clear

It is eminently desirable to prevent accidents and mental illness, to reduce the numbers of teenage conceptions and those infected by the HIV virus, but the means by which these targets are to be achieved are not spelt out. Health education, if it works, might achieve the targets for sexual health but for accidents, legislation to improve home and road design would seem to be essential. Exactly how it is hoped to reduce the number of suicides is a mystery. The inclusion of these targets in the report would appear to be rhetorical.

Category three: not achievable

Reduction of coronary heart disease primarily by changes in the diet will not work because the link between diet and heart disease fails to fulfil Bradford Hill's canons of epidemiological proof.

Even with this restricted list of targets for prevention and the most optimistic forecasts, the overall net effect on the health of the nation will quite clearly be modest.

Prevention as a strategy for promoting health is limited by our scientific understanding of the causation of disease and the logistical problems – whether to do with screening or health education – of translating those targets into practice. So, though the two great projects of medicine – the preventive and the therapeutic – are in theory complementary, prevention is not a substitute for the therapeutic, and a health strategy that suggests otherwise is misleading.

The need for caution in interpreting low level risks reported by epidemiologists

Peter Lee

Introduction

Hardly a week goes by without a newspaper article reporting that some aspect of everyday life allegedly leads to an increased risk of yet another disease. There are a number of reasons why there is a need for considerable caution in interpreting these findings, particularly when the claimed increase in risk is by a relatively small factor. For example, the link between lung cancer and passive smoking, which I have studied in depth, and to which I will refer in more detail, is an instance where incautious and possibly incorrect claims have been made due to a failure to take into account the limitations of epidemiology. Such inadequately justified claims of risk result in the public being needlessly worried, but there are ways in which this menace can be combatted and these will also be considered.

Epidemiology and types of epidemiological study

Epidemiology is the examination of relationships between a putative causative agent and a disease by observing human populations. This can be done in a variety of ways, of which the most common are the *prospective* and the *case-control* study. In the prospective (or longitudinal or cohort) study, information on exposure to the agent (and other relevant risk factors) is collected from subjects who are initially disease-free and a comparison is made between the subsequent rates of onset of the disease or death in groups with different levels of exposure. To obtain enough cases of the disease for the relationship with exposure to be assessed accurately may involve large numbers followed up over a considerable period of time. It is for this reason that many epidemiologists prefer to use the case-control study in which current and past exposure to the agent in a group of patients with the disease is compared to that in a control group without the disease. The control group should be representative, in terms of exposure, of the population from which the diseased patients arose.

Other types of epidemiological study include *cross-sectional* and *ecological* studies. In the cross-sectional study a sample of the population is taken at one point in time and data on exposure and presence of disease are recorded. In the ecological study data on average exposure and average risk are obtained for a number of different populations, for example in different countries, and an attempt is made to ascertain whether average risk varies according to average exposure.

Problems in interpreting epidemiological data
There are a number of theoretical reasons why an association may be observed between an agent and a disease other than the simple reason that the agent causes the disease.

Chance: where a study is carried out to test a hypothesis which has been clearly defined in advance, standard statistical techniques are available to compute the probability (p) of the observed result occurring, given no true effect of the agent. While some epidemiologists use $p = 0.05$ as a cut-off, treating lower levels as statistically significant and therefore 'proof' of the hypothesis, others regard p values less than 0.001 as very convincing evidence of an association, p values in the range 0.01–0.001 as quite convincing, and p values in the range 0.1–0.01 as suggestive.

Where no hypothesis was clearly defined in advance, one

must obviously be wary in interpreting these p values. In a large prospective study, there will be data on hundreds of risk factors and deaths will be caused by a range of diseases. With so many possible combinations of risk factors and diseases, and the ability of modern computers rapidly to investigate all combinations, it is only to be expected that statistical analysis will throw up a whole number of new associations which are 'significant' but which have, in fact, arisen purely by chance.

Publication bias: there is a general proposition that when assessing an association, one should use *all* the available data. This is a sound enough idea but the reviewer has to be particularly wary of the likelihood that 'all published data' is not the same thing as 'all the data that exists'. Numerous papers have now demonstrated the dangers of what is known as 'publication bias', resulting from the fact that studies showing a statistically significant relationship are more likely to be published than those that do not. Often an author may not bother to submit a paper unless it shows a statistically significant relationship and if he does try to submit a paper showing no relationship between the agent and the disease in question, a journal may be loth to accept it, regarding it as uninteresting to its readers.

Reverse causation: just because there is consistent and highly significant evidence of an association between an agent and a disease does not necessarily imply that the agent causes the disease. It is possible that the causal process was in the reverse direction. Thus evidence that more subjects with chronic bronchitis gave up smoking in the previous year than was the case for healthy controls, does not imply that giving up smoking increases the chance of getting chronic bronchitis. Rather it reflects the fact that people who have chronic bronchitis are particularly likely to give up smoking.

Similarly, the increased death rate from stomach cancer in people taking the anti-ulcer drug, cimetidine, does not prove that cimetidine causes stomach cancer but rather that stomach cancer was initially misdiagnosed as stomach ulcer which was the reason why the patient took cimetidine in the first place.

Misclassification of exposure: random errors in determining exposure tend to dilute any true relationship with the disease. However, errors may not be random. Knowledge of, or indeed presence of, the disease may affect recall of exposure and cause a spurious relationship. For example, an association between cancer and family history of that cancer may arise, not because of a genetic effect, but because cases with cancer may be more aware of other similar cancers in the family than cancer-free controls who would have had less reason to discuss cancer with relatives. Note that such 'recall bias' should not arise in prospective studies.

Misclassification of diagnosis: random misclassification of diagnosis also tends to dilute a true relationship of an agent with a disease. Again, differential misclassification may, however, produce a false-positive relationship. In a study of necropsies in which primary lung cancer was found, it was shown that the diagnosis was much more likely to have been made in-life if the patient smoked than if he did not. The reason, of course, was that his doctor knew of the well-publicised relationship of smoking with lung cancer and he was therefore more suspicious that lung cancer might be present if the patient smoked. He was therefore more likely to have conducted the appropriate tests than if a non-smoking patient had presented with similar symptoms. In this situation the bias resulted in an overestimation of the strength of the relationship of smoking to lung cancer.

Confounding: in *experimental* studies, where subjects are randomly assigned to exposure, the groups differ only in respect of exposure to the agent under investigation, and do not differ systematically in respect of exposure to other agents which may have bearing on the disease in question. In *epi-*

demiological studies, however, there is no randomisation and allowances must be made for the possibility that an observed association between an agent and a disease may result from what is termed confounding by the effects of another agent (or agents).

There are numerous examples of false associations due to confounding. For example, in a recent study comparing heavy smokers with lifelong non-smokers in respect of the presence of 33 factors generally considered to be associated with an adverse effect on health, it was observed that the heavy smokers were significantly worse off in respect of no less than 27 of these (*inter alia* they were less educated, of lower social class, worked more often in occupations with a cancer risk, drank more alcohol and coffee, ate more fatty and fried foods, ate less fresh fruit and vegetables, slept less, and did nothing to keep healthy) and were only better off in respect of two (they were less likely to be obese and to eat sweet foods). Furthermore, it was interesting to note that, among those who had never smoked, living with a smoker was clearly associated with many of these adverse risk factors. It was evident that these differences in risk factor prevalence were capable, if not taken into account, of distorting the relationship of both passive smoking and smoking with a range of diseases.

Confounding is unlikely to explain very strong observed relationships but it is a very important consideration when observed relative risks are only modest. In the case of the association between marriage to a smoker and lung cancer which, it is claimed, indicates that passive smoking causes the disease, one is talking of a relative risk estimated to be only about 1.1 to 1.3, which could easily have arisen as a result of confounding. A number of researchers have estimated the bias due to confounding by diet alone to exceed 1.1 (marriage to a smoker is associated with increased consumption of dietary fat and reduced consumption of fresh fruit and vegetables both known correlates of lung cancer risk).

Of course, epidemiologists often try to take confounding factors into account in their analyses and there are established statistical techniques for doing this. These produce what are termed 'adjusted risk estimates' and, where there is a single, clearly defined 'confounder' which has been accurately measured, they can be quite straightforward. But unless data for all relevant confounders have been collected and considered, the adjusted relative risk estimate may still be biased. The problem is that for many diseases the major causes are simply not yet known, and these unknown causes may be associated with the agent of interest, so causing confounding.

Inaccuracy in measurement of confounding variables is another reason why attempts to adjust for confounding may fail. Various authors have made it clear that statistical techniques which adjust for an inaccurately measured variable do not remove the full confounding effect of that variable and leave what is referred to as 'residual confounding', the magnitude of which can be quite substantial. It is unfortunately true that many agents are difficult to quantify precisely. Thus, measuring social class is an imprecise measure of specific occupational risk factors; dietary questionnaires provide an imprecise measure of consumption of specific foods, nutrients or vitamins; while questions on number of sexual partners may not only be answered inaccurately, but may inaccurately quantify exposure to sexually transmitted infections which may be the underlying causes of certain diseases. An example of a reported association which may well be spurious, despite the fact that it has been seen in many studies, is that between smoking and cervical cancer. There is abundant evidence that cervical cancer is caused by a sexually transmitted virus, and also evidence that smokers have many more sexual partners than non-smokers and are thus more at risk of exposure to the virus. Although adjustment in analysis for the reported number of sexual partners does not eliminate the association of smoking with cervical cancer, the reduced association may

41

well simply reflect 'residual confounding' and does not, therefore, demonstrate that smoking causes the disease.

Biases due to selection: the population studied should be
representative of the population to whom inferences are to be
made. People who agree to be interviewed or who reply to
mailed questionnaires may be untypical, in respect of exposure and disease, of those who do not. Studies where data
for cases and controls are collected by differing procedures
with differing response rates, eg cases interviewed in hospital
directly, controls interviewed at home by telephone, are
particularly open to selection bias.

When the study requires that only a specified sub-set of the
population be considered, bias may arise if some subjects enter
the study in error. A good example of this is in studies of passive
smoking and lung cancer. These are typically conducted among
lifelong never-smokers (to try to avoid problems of confounding by effect of active smoking) and compare risk in subjects
married to smokers and to non-smokers. The problem arises
because a proportion of current or past smokers deny having
smoked when interviewed and they will have a relatively much
higher risk of lung cancer than those who truly have never
smoked. Because smokers are more than averagely likely to
marry smokers, it results in a higher proportion of misclassified
'ever' smokers among the 'never' smokers married to smokers
than among those married to non-smokers. There is a difference of opinion as to the extent of bias resulting from this
source, but it certainly is an important reason why one should
have grave doubts about interpreting the slight increase in risk
of lung cancer in non-smoking women married to smokers as
indicating any effect of ETS exposure.

Consistency: apart from a need to consider various types of bias,
it is also necessary to be sure that all the facts fit together
consistently. For example, active smoking is much more
strongly associated with risk of the squamous-cell lung cancer

than with the other common form, adenocarcinoma. It would be expected then, if passive smoking did cause lung cancer, it would be of the squamous-cell type. It is interesting to note however, that the evidence here is quite conflicting. Of 14 studies that sought to make the distinction, four included data more consistent with a relationship between passive smoking and squamous-cell cancer; another four found a relationship with adenocarcinoma, one found a relationship with both types, and the remainder found no relationship with either type.

How do we get more reliable conclusions?
Although epidemiology has certainly been of value in demonstrating the importance of a number of factors in the aetiology of various diseases, it is clear that some of its conclusions cannot really be trusted. Where an observed association is very strong, there are reasonable grounds for concluding it could not have resulted from chance or from one of the various forms of bias present in epidemiological studies. Where an association is weak, however, these alternative interpretations can be excluded only with difficulty. Even now it is rare that one can be sure that a reported 50 per cent increase in risk (ie, a relative risk of 1.5) is genuine, which is unfortunate since, for many common diseases and exposures, an agent causing a 50 per cent increase in risk might be very important.

What improvements could be made to get more reliable conclusions? Though there is probably no way in which we could ever reliably detect increases below a relative risk of 1.05 or 1.1, there are a number of measures that could be taken to make studies more sensitive.

It would be an advantage if journals considering papers for publication were to demand sight of a copy of the study protocol, which would make it clear precisely what was done and why. This would not only make it evident to the journal when a paper was presenting a finding which resulted from 'data-dredging', rather than testing a prior hypothesis, but would also make any limitations of the study clearer.

Epidemiologists should be encouraged to do better studies with an emphasis on:

- *Using appropriate control groups:* controls with diseases that may be caused by the agent of interest are inappropriate, as are controls from different hospitals with different catchment areas.

- *Collecting data from cases and controls in a comparable manner:* answers may depend on the circumstances of interview or on the respondent (subject or next-of-kin) and this should be the same for cases and controls.

- *Collecting data blind:* where possible diagnosis should be carried out without knowledge of the patient's exposure history, and data on exposure and other variables should be collected without knowledge of the diagnosis.

- *Collecting data on many potential confounding variables:* there are still studies which appear to collect no data at all on any potential confounders.

- *Getting high response rates:* techniques such as mailed questionnaires, which usually produce a low rate of response are not ideal. Direct interviews, with multiple approaches if the subject is not initially available for interview, are better.

- *Getting complete follow-up:* there have been prospective studies in US states which made no attempt to detect deaths occurring in other states, let alone in other countries. People who move are atypical of people who stay put in many respects.

- *Getting data on accuracy of key variables:* unless one has some idea of how accurately key variables are determined, it may be impossible to interpret the findings. It is useful therefore, where possible, to obtain repeat measurements from the same source and/or from independent sources.

In interpreting the results of a study, epidemiologists should also be much more aware that an association between a disease and an agent can only be regarded as evidence of a cause-and-effect relationship if *all* alternative explanations can be ruled out. They should also try to be aware of *all* relevant data from other studies. To aid this, it would be useful to set up more organisations like the Oxford Group (which conducts meta-analyses of data from randomised clinical trials on a number of topics). They not only ask the authors of published papers to provide their data on computer, to allow more appropriate combined analyses to be conducted, but they also write to scientists, who they believe may have conducted unpublished studies on the subject, to obtain their data.

Another aid to epidemiology would be to start a really large prospective study on a representative sample of perhaps one or two million people in which data would be collected on a wide variety of risk factors. It should be feasible to obtain both government and private-sector funding for such a project which, over the years, would provide good data on the relationship of various risk factors to numerous causes of death. By ensuring that all the study findings, significant or otherwise, are available (either in monographs or through computer-accessible files) such a study could authoritatively act to counter numerous unreliable reports of associations based on small case-control studies.

Finally, there should be a better relationship between epidemiologists and medical journalists, to assist in explaining the limitations of their discipline to the general public. Epidemiology is capable of making valuable discoveries, but it will lose its credibility unless more attempts are made to ensure that its findings, as reported in the media, actually are meaningful.

Health promotion and NHS reform: a critique of *Health of the Nation*

Bruce Charlton

Introduction

Health of the Nation[1] is a major strategic plan intended to improve the general level of health in England – similar documents apply to Scotland and Wales. One of the stated goals of these White Papers is to effect a significant shift in provision of health services in favour of health promotion.[2] This amounts to a transfer of scarce health resources away from care of the sick and towards services for the healthy. The process could end by damaging health, diminishing public satisfaction and encouraging wholesale government interference in everyday life. Therefore the limitations of *Health of the Nation* both define, and are defined by, the 'limits of prevention'.

I should first make it clear that *Health of the Nation* is, of course, well-intentioned, but unfortunately misguided. It recalls Bernard Shaw's wise remark: 'the path to Hell is paved with good intentions'. Living as we do, in an era when politics seems unappealing and ineffective, the wide perspective and galloping optimism of *Health of the Nation* may strike people as alluring. But a sceptic might ask how a Government which so notably fails to attain legitimate political targets in foreign policy, law and order, and management of the economy can hope to deliver the transformation in health and well-being promised by the White Paper.

The ambition is, indeed, breathtaking. What is proposed is a programme of social change which will comprehensively reshape the life of every citizen, and transform the whole way in which medicine is practised and health services are delivered.

A managed health service

Health of the Nation can be interpreted as the latest attempt by government to get control of the NHS. The aim is a managed health service, with managers in control; whereas in the past we had merely an administered health service, with nobody in control – or at any rate no single group of workers.

After the 1974 'reforms' the National Health Service had become an immovable mass, jammed tight with committees who were expert at preventing change. The 1983 Management Inquiry by Roy Griffiths[3] was followed by the introduction of general managers, who were given the power to run things, and were made responsible if things did not run. But how could the health service be managed when most of the actual work was carried out by semi-autonomous professional groups such as doctors, nurses and other health workers? Managers might be able to influence the structures and the money, and carry through plans to the level of the health professional, but they were stopped short at the relationship between the health professional and the patient.

The use of 'target-setting' can be seen as a managerial strategy for influencing autonomous groups in situations where behaviour cannot directly be prescribed, 'so that each part of the NHS can be actively managed, monitored and improved'.[4] Managers do not yet instruct clinicians how to treat each individual patient, but target-setting can ensure that patient-doctor interactions take place within defined boundaries.

Target-setting has been adopted as the main instrument for strategic planning in the NHS. So it is reasonable to ask what it

47

means to set 'targets' for health. After all, any mistakes in this 'five year plan' style of managing are likely to have serious adverse consequences. The resemblance between *Health of the Nation* and a Soviet-style command economy should alert us to the dangers of a monolithic approach to national planning.

Targets or objectives?
A target is something which should be hit, whereas an objective shows in which direction we should be aiming. Some of the targets set by *Health of the Nation* can more plausibly be interpreted as objectives or priority areas.

Altering priorities will tend adversely to affect non-targeted areas. These are the 'opportunity costs' – some other activity must be curtailed to allow new priorities to be addressed. Non-targeted areas will suffer unless extra resources are created (or unless overall efficiency is improved). Hitting the target must therefore compensate for the disadvantages of neglecting other areas.

Unfortunately we do not know how to hit all the targets: either they have not been properly thought through, or else they are not 'real' targets. Although *Health of the Nation* is composed of numerous seemingly authoritative statements, many of these are actually controversial or misleading, as for example, the supposed 'link' between sunburn and malignant melanoma. The confident style papers over a great deal of scientific uncertainty. For instance, the whole strategy of classical 'health education' has been powerfully challenged in the research literature – it may be ineffective or even counter-productive in some cases, as when advertising campaigns to reduce drug addiction actually seem to make the problem worse.

Health of the Nation gives the impression that much more is known about the cause, prevention and cure of sickness than is really the case. A good deal is, indeed, known about the effects of cigarette smoking, and it has been well established that modifying the level of smoking will modify the risk of various diseases such as lung cancer, coronary heart disease and stroke. Smoking is thus a true 'risk factor'. But the same does not apply to alcohol consumption, diet and exercise, except at the extremes (heavy, sustained drinking, massive obesity and a totally sedentary life are certainly bad for health – but their relationship to sickness at more normal levels is much less clear). Further, to assume without experimental evidence that reducing or removing a risk factor will prevent the associated disease is an elementary mistake; yet this mistake is made throughout the White Paper.

Targets have other dangers. Reducing the overall suicide rate in the population, and also suicides among the mentally ill, are goals which we do not know how to achieve at present; neither are we on the verge of a breakthrough. The White Paper admits that 'the contributory causes of suicide are by no means fully understood'.[5] Why, then is suicide-reduction an official and quantified target (the only one for mental health)? If health service managers, on performance-related contracts, try to meet such targets without knowing how, there is considerable potential for wasted efforts and bad outcomes. Indeed, there may be a temptation to achieve targets by massaging the statistics rather than through modifying practice.

Perhaps we should interpret the exhortations to reduce suicide rates in the light of being objectives rather than targets: as attempting to improve the clinical management of severe depression which, although probably accounting for only about a half of all suicides, is an important cause. The suicide rate is thus being used as a very crude barometer of the effectiveness of psychiatric services for depression. It is hard to imagine how such an inaccurate measure can possibly lead to improved management.

More worryingly, target-setting may be nothing but a public relations exercise – a method of advertising that the Government is non-specifically 'concerned' about a problem – perhaps also a method of defusing hostile criticism by pretending that something concrete is being done. The extent to which sheer wishful thinking permeates the White Paper causes one to suspect that there is a sense in which the document is itself intended to stand as a symbol for idealistic and caring government.

Positive and negative targets

The *Health of the Nation* strategy talks only in terms of improvements in health services. Yet the political reality is that the health service will have finite and fixed resources. Level-funding is the likely future. Health provision is therefore a zero-sum game: improvements in one area will only be at the cost of cuts in other areas.

The White Paper proposes investment in positively-targeted areas but there is no mention of cuts in provision or 'disinvestment'. This evasion is understandable from a political perspective. Selecting only positive targets may be dishonest (or at least disingenuous), but it is a powerful rhetorical device. Critics of the White Paper are placed in the position of arguing *against* providing extra resources for patient groups who are, no doubt, very deserving.

So where will extra resources to attain the targets come from? The usual answer is that resources can be generated by efficiency gains (which generally means getting fewer people to work harder for less money). However, even if this can be done, it usually happens that any such savings are more than swallowed up by the increased administrative costs of introducing a new system. Money has then merely been transferred from medical services to the salaries of administrators and managers.

Hoping that improvements can be paid for out of efficiency gains is not sensible. Improving an organisation as complex as the health service is very difficult and results in a multitude of 'unforeseen consequences'. Making the NHS more efficient is equally hard. Both cost money – at least in the short-term. Attempting to improve the health service and also make it more efficient, at the same time, and with only level funding, is not just difficult – it is impossible. This policy is doomed to fail.

Shirking the duty to identify negative targets represents an expensive, as well as damaging, failure of political nerve. Because, while positive targets inevitably cost money, negative targets might actually save money. If, for instance, areas of ineffective or inappropriate health service provision could confidently be identified (for example, 'counsellors' employed in general pratices), then cuts could liberate resources for investment in other aspects of health service work – without damaging health service provision. The result might be a leaner and fitter NHS, instead of a weaker and feebler one.

Two rival philosophies of reform

Health of the Nation must also be seen in relation to the other NHS 'reforms'. Here there is a clear conflict: two distinct, and perhaps incompatible, philosophies of what the NHS is, and what it should be.

One view sees the NHS as a giant organisation: as if it were a 'company' producing health. The problem is how most efficiently to organise this company: the method is essentially one of organisation theory. The other view sees the NHS not as one company, but as a massive market place: an arena where a multitude of smaller interests compete for resources. The problem in this case is how to ensure fair competition: the method is through internal markets.

The *Health of the Nation* embodies a 'corporate' philosophy. It conceptualises the NHS as a massive organisation, and its solutions are essentially bureaucratic. The resemblance between *Health of the Nation* and the 'rationalistic' world of classical 'scientific socialism' is too obvious to escape comment. The White Paper's emphasis on grand central planning (albeit after 'consultation') is reminiscent of the simple certainties of a bygone era: those wartime propaganda pamphlets promising a sunny future of gleaming-white concrete high-rise homes set amidst the fields, by-passes and industrial estates of carefully planned 'New Towns' . . . Its supporters can see themselves as the knights in shining armour who will transform England into a green and pleasant (and tobacco-free) land.

The other group of NHS reforms (principally the 1989 document, *Working for Patients*[6]) come from a different world entirely: the radical libertarianism of the 'New Right'. This sees the NHS as, ideally, a marketplace. The thrust of New Right thinking has been to abandon rational planning as a bad job, and focus instead upon increasing competition (especially 'internal markets') as the means of achieving a more effective, efficient and responsive health service. This tendency sees a multiplication of semi-autonomous Fund-holding General Practices and Trust Hospitals as 'the jewels in the crown' of the new NHS.

It is difficult to imagine how two such opposed reforming tendencies can ever be brought into harmony. On the one side we have the corporate vision of a centrally-directed, top-down national initiative: a pyramid which stretches from the Department of Health at the top, through Regional and District tiers down to the multitude of doctor-patient interactions at the base. (Or, to be accurate, the multitude of 'health-care-worker and service-user interactions'.) On the other side we have Fund-holding General Practices and Trust Hospitals battling it out in some version of Adam Smith's marketplace (Health Authorities having been abolished somewhere along the way). On the one hand we have the notion that high quality services and rational decision-making should be imposed and regulated by bureaucratic procedures. On the other hand is the idea that salvation lies in consumer power: with the 'invisible hand' of the market summating a multitude of purchaser preferences to conjure up appropriate services from health providers.

The politics of health

But neither the *Health of the Nation* strategy and its ideal of a managed health service, nor the marketplace strategy and its ideal of a consumer-friendly NHS, are likely to improve health care. Both philosophies are fundamentally adversarial – pitting different interest groups against one another, and taking a cynical view of human motivations. Both strategies are utopian, reductionist and ideological – based on ideas of what 'ought' to work, rather than developing from what actually does work. Both try to ignore the qualities of the individuals involved, and imagine a 'human-proof' health service. And both are anti-institutional.

Having criticised the politics of NHS reforms, I must here say something of what I would prefer and why. I prefer a more traditional view of British political life, starting from where we are and what we are, a view which allows an important role for existing institutions and practices. Institutions mediate between the state and the citizen, and ensure that the individual does not stand alone. Individuals are, indeed, largely formed and protected by society's institutions, and are dependent upon them for their freedom and happiness.

Without institutions the citizen is merely a commodity in the marketplace and a pawn in the political system. Fortunately, institutions are resilient: they have their own purposes, powers and privileges granted over time, and are usually valued and supported by those who understand them. Nonetheless they are more easily destroyed than created, and more easily impaired than improved. Against the tide, I wish to see institutions reformed rather than swept aside. In a time of change I suspect that they are our best hope for the future; the future not just of the NHS and medical practice, but of the country at large. At their best they are 'human-sized', give meaning to life, and constitute the 'checks and balances' which help prevent democracy from degenerating into elective dictatorship.

The way forward lies in reducing regulations and bureaucracy and minimising market incentives. Instead we should nurture professional self-regulation and encourage high standards and an *ethos* of service. Privileges are allowed in return for responsibilities. Those who abuse their privileges must be swiftly detected and disciplined – but little else is required in terms of external control. In other words, the simplest, cheapest and best way to run a health service is by relearning the art of trusting professionals to get on with their jobs.

I fear the relentless 'politicisation' of the NHS and its activities, so that politics comes to affect every person who works in the health service and not merely its managers. This amounts to the contamination of the NHS and medicine by political expediency. And this process moves our society further towards the kind of 'totalitarian' state where politics is inescapable and countervailing power has been neutralised (although, thank heavens, we still have a long way to go!).

In looking at the conflict between the two philosophies of NHS reform – between markets and management, between the competitive and the corporate ethic – we might predict that planning will win. Governments can control civil servants more easily by line management than by competition, and markets must inevitably be regulated. Also the consequences of markets might prove politically unpalatable, making interference a certainty. We will probably end up getting the worst of both worlds – the expense and unwieldiness of a 'pretend' market system, operating within a rigid and equally expensive bureaucratic framework: no significant improvement at the cost of much more administration.

But maybe stability is not wanted by those who run the NHS. After all, there are management theorists who argue that chaos is desirable for a thriving organisation. It could be that a state of *permanent*, chaos is intended for the NHS. *Health of the Nation* provides a conduit for feeding an unending stream of priorities and initiatives into the system, to keep us all 'on our toes'. Again a similarity with communist notions of a 'permanent revolution' suggests itself. I strongly doubt that this would be conducive to good health care, whatever its virtues in big business or utopian politics. But we see here that peculiar radical alliance between the free-marketeering right wing and the revolutionary left wing which has characterised so much of modern political debate.

Health of the Nation, despite its up-to-date rhetoric and the verbal concessions it makes to local flexibility, is merely an example of old-fashioned 'rational' social engineering, of a kind which has been tried and failed many times before. The attempt to promote health 'in its widest sense' is partly utopian rhetoric and partly an attempt to pursue a political agenda by other means. Of course the White Paper does have its good points – certainly it has led to some interesting debate, and some of its recommendations are sensible. However, on the whole, *Health of the Nation* has blurred the issues rather than clarified them, and under the guise of health promotion it has extended the limits of preventive medicine to include most of life.

As for improvements in the health service – if we can manage them, and that will not be easy – they will come from a complex and constant process of multiple initiatives and negotiations. The hope is to preserve the benefits of past practice while trying to discard only the deficiencies. This is a gradual and difficult process: there are no shortcuts to excellence.

Prevention and clinical freedom: a clinician's view

John Hampton

Introduction

The main achievement of the NHS reforms which separate purchasers and providers will not be improved efficiency or cost reduction: it will be the acceptance and admission that everything has its cost, that resources are finite, and that overt choices have to be made. Covert choices have, of course, been made for many years, but mainly on a basis of muddle, fudge and long waiting lists. Health care has always been rationed whatever the system. In a free market system, as in the USA, the rationing depends on the individual's ability to pay the insurance premiums, and the result is that millions are un-protected. In a socialised system, such as the NHS, resources are limited by the proportion of the tax base allocated to health, and until now the theory has been that everything is possible – but the individual may have to wait. Covert ration-ing comes in when doctors adjust their concept of what the patient needs according to what is available. If as a result of the NHS reforms we start talking about choice rather than ration-ing, much will have been achieved.

Once we do start talking about choices, we can see straight away that a choice will have to be made between prevention and treatment. Prevention is not simply a cheap alternative to treatment. Preventing a case of most diseases costs as much or more than treating the effects of that disease in an individual patient, and while it is clearly desirable that disease should not exist, it is less obvious that a healthy individual with a low risk of disease will be prepared to pay much to have that risk lowered a little further. The trouble with the prevention strategy as set out in *Health of the Nation* is that it makes a great play of setting targets for health, without considering the likelihood of success, the cost, or the cost in terms of lost opportunities. It lacks an honest admission that we know too little about the causes of most diseases to be confident we can prevent them. What we now need is a critical appraisal of the chances that any individual preventive measure will work, the cost of preventing (or more properly, deferring) a single death, the appropriateness of the measure, and the means by which a choice to implement that measure will be made.

Prevention: effectiveness and cost
First, then, the effectiveness of prevention: if we cannot do everything, then we must be sure that those things we do are effective. We have no hesitation in acknowledging that treatments must be proved effective before they are accepted, and there is no reason why prevention should not be subject to the same stringency. In a few areas this has been achieved. For example, we know from the first MRC Hypertension Trial that, by treating 850 patients with mild hypertension for a year, one stroke can be prevented. We also know the effects of screening for cervical and breast cancer. Such examples, however, result from active intervention in high risk individuals. Such evidence as there is suggests that most routine screening procedures involving the whole population achieve little, and such screening is performed both at financial expense and at the expense of alarm among those who are screened. Above all, there is little point in screening when it is unproved that action is beneficial. Here the classic example must be the blood cholesterol level, where so far it has been impossible to prove that its reduction actually reduces the death rate.

The costs of screening are dealt with elsewhere but suffice to say that, while some calculations are easy – for example, the cost per life saved by installing a mile of motorway crash barrier, or of making the cabs of tractors safe in the event of an accident – in many cases they are far more difficult. The major problem is to distinguish between screening and preventive action in high risk individuals (tractor drivers, those with a bad family history of hypertension, heart disease or breast cancer) and taking action on a population basis without worrying about individuals at all. There is now reasonably convincing evidence that a low blood cholesterol level carries an increased risk, so reducing the average cholesterol level in the whole population may have two balancing effects: those who start with a high cholesterol level and therefore have a high coronary risk might possibly benefit by achieving normal cholesterol levels, while those who start with a normal level may have their risk of non-coronary diseases increased if their plasma cholesterol level is reduced by too much. Since the basis of population manipulation is that no measurements are made, there is no way of telling which individuals might benefit and which might be harmed. While it might be possible to monitor and attribute changes in death rates from coronary disease from such a programme, it would be far more difficult to calculate the costs of less clear-cut effects such as an increase in assorted cancers and depressive illnesses which are not so easy to identify as heart attacks, but which might result from an attempt to change the mean cholesterol level of the population.

Prevention and appropriateness
We must, then, be sure that what we do is appropriate both to our needs and to our knowledge. 'Appropriateness' started off as a medical term, but it has now been highjacked by others – in particular by lay people and by politicians.

For a doctor, the best definition of appropriateness is perhaps that developed by the RAND corporation:

> An intervention is appropriate when the Health benefit (mortality, morbidity, etc) exceeds the negative consequences (risks, pain, etc) by a sufficient margin to make the intervention worth doing.

Much has been done to define and quantify medical appropriateness, which in the main depends upon the identification of hard evidence of treatment efficacy, and where hard evidence is lacking, by using reasonably scientific techniques for codifying expert opinion.

On the other hand, the lay view of appropriateness is quite different. The definition used by a Department of Health Working Party on research into appropriateness was:

> Appropriate care is the intervention most likely to produce the outcome desired by the individual patient.

There will be a difference of attitude to appropriateness between those who either have the disease in question themselves or have a relative with it, when all sorts of high-tech investigations into treatment will be considered appropriate, and those who are healthy and have had no personal experience of the disease. Such people will take a more sceptical view, with an eye on their tax return.

The third view of appropriateness, that of society as a whole, has two elements. First, there is the social conscience which has to decide how far to provide for those who are unable to help themselves, and whose voices are not heard. Second, someone has to decide on the proportion of the tax base which is to be committed to health care. The absolute size of the tax base is probably more important than the proportion devoted to health, but both this and the distribution of tax revenue can only be decided at a political level, and ultimately through the ballot box. In this crucial sense, and as pointed out by Virchow many years ago, medicine cannot and should not be separated from politics.

Prevention and choice

How then are choices to be made? Doctors will always shroud-wave in support of their own particular speciality, as will patients and those with affected friends and relatives. Surveys have shown that healthy laymen rate hospitals and sophisticated medicine highly, but give psychiatric disease and the care of very low birth weight babies a low priority. Much depends, as in all referenda, on the precise wording of the question asked.

The Dutch Government has commissioned an infinitely more thoughtful and valuable publication than *Health of the Nation*. Entitled *Choices in Health Care*, it accepts that in a world of finite resources choices will have to be made, and to some extent it covers the same ground as the Department of Health Working Party Document on Appropriateness. The Dutch conclusion is that 'rationing' health care is politically unacceptable, and that the basis of governmental intervention must be to care for those who cannot help themselves, whatever the public view of the appropriateness of such an action. The report suggests that medical treatment should be put in a list in priority order, and a line drawn through that list at whatever point marks the limits of funds available. Conditions or procedures below that line will be excluded from the basic package of health care that must be available to all.

The State of Oregon in the USA has attempted to put such a system into operation, but we shall have to wait and see whether or not it can be made to work here. Central to discussions relating to choice must be the premise that something that does not work can never be appropriate. Where does prevention fit into the debate? If we have an important disease where a measure of proven effectiveness can be introduced so that the cost of preventing a single case of the disease can be calculated and shown to be comparable to the cost of symptomatic relief in a patient with an established disease (for example, hip replacement), then presumably that preventive measure will be accepted in the health-care package. If it does not meet these criteria, logic suggests that it should not be implemented.

Prevention and politics
Several chapters in this book have suggested that preventive policies go too *far*; too far, that is, for the scientific evidence or too far in infringement of individual liberty. There is also a chance that they do not go far *enough*; far enough, that is, to be effective and that going far enough will take them well beyond the confines of the Department of Health and the current *Health of the Nation* plan. The case is based on the generally agreed fact that the main improvements in health over the centuries have come not from medical care, but from improvements in the socio-economic status of the population. The most important marker for later ill health for an individual is to be in Social Class V, among whose members there is a reduction in life expectancy of eight years, compared with those in Social Class I. To being in Social Class V we must now add the ill health known to be associated with unemployment. Raising the housing and education standards of those in Social Class V, and reducing unemployment, is the responsibility respectively of the Departments of the Environment, Education and Employment, not the Department of Health.

The greatest improvement in health that could now be obtained in the UK by a single preventive measure would be to abolish smoking: this could probably be achieved through a package of tax increases, advertising bans, and prevention of smoking in public places – but all this, it would appear, is a matter for the Treasury and the Party Chairman, who guesses at the likely effects of such actions on votes in the next election. It would appear that there is little that the Department of Health can or will do about smoking, and this seriously questions the whole attitude of that Department to the prevention of disease. The inescapable conclusion is that disease prevention should be taken out of the hands of the Department of Health, which should be left to concentrate on disease treatment. Other relevant Departments should perhaps have their budgets increased specifically to deal with the promotion of health. Whether one thinks current policy goes too far or not far enough, it is apparent that its current formulation satisfies neither view. Instead it manages to combine being intrusive and ineffective.

Prevention and clinical freedom
All this leaves the doctor in a difficult position. His duty lies with his individual patient, for whom he must do whatever he considers to be in his or her best interests. This is commonly described as clinical freedom. Clinical freedom, however, already has considerable limitations. There are the social standards which change from time to time but are reflected in law (for example, abortion) and the law now gives patients apparent rights by charter. Doctors are limited professionally by their competence and accreditation through professional bodies, and this is ultimately controlled by malpractice suits in the Courts. At a slightly more subtle level, doctors' actions are constrained by the availability of resources and by their responsibility to other patients: doctors know that if, for example, they refer an 85 year-old for a heart valve replacement, a 45 year-old who needs a coronary bypass graft operation will be pushed further down the waiting list. Quite properly doctors' actions are limited by peer pressure, now being codified by audit, and by the increasingly widespread use of treatment protocols and guidelines. In theory – but as we all know, not in practice – a doctor's clinical practice is not affected by NHS funding.

If we now see preventive medicine as just another form of 'treatment', different only in that it is healthy subjects who are being 'treated' and not patients with established disease, prevention can be seen as just another choice. A doctor's clinical freedom to treat a patient will be limited still further if a significant proportion of the health-care budget is devoted to disease prevention. The appropriateness of prevention depends primarily on its proven effectiveness, but after that we will have to accept that different groups will see its appropriateness differently. Doctors are sometimes accused of being 'against' prevention as if it might reduce their power and income. In fact, doctors should see it as a clinical freedom to speak firmly against preventive measures that seem a poor choice in comparison with treating patients who have established disease.

High blood cholesterol: a problem with no ready solution

L E Ramsay, W W Yeo, P R Jackson

Introduction

Even those with little interest in health matters will be aware there are widely differing views among experts on the problem of cholesterol, and what should be done about it. A major factor in this is the diverse background of these experts – some are cholesterol specialists, some epidemiologists, some public health experts, some cardiologists – and all tend to view the problem as it presents to their particular speciality. We have been drawn, or even forced, into this controversial area only very recently, approaching the cholesterol problem as general physicians with an interest in rational therapeutics, and with extensive clinical and research experience in high blood pressure (hypertension), a condition which has much in common with high cholesterol.

Medicine and the individual

As general physicians our every day work is with individual patients, who want to know what is wrong with them, what is to be done about it, and what the outcome will be. When it comes to prevention they are interested in their individual risk, what benefit they themselves will get from treatment, and how much inconvenience, discomfort and risk they will have to accept to get this benefit. They are not interested in the mortality and morbidity statistics for England and Wales, but only in the personal contribution they may make to these statistics. Moreover, with a few notable exceptions, they prefer to have nothing to do with doctors if they can possibly avoid it.

Rational therapeutics

Nowadays an interest in therapeutics means an interest in controlled clinical trials. With rare exceptions these provide the only true measure of the worth of a treatment – an unbiased and unconfounded measure of its benefit, and of its cost in terms of inconvenience, subjective side-effects and serious adverse effects. Having an interest in the management of hypertension, we have watched a series of large long-term outcome trials of hypertension treatment unfold over three decades, which have explored the benefits and risks of treatment, and have encompassed severe, moderate and mild high blood pressure; old and young people; men and women; white and black people; and comparisons of one type of drug treatment versus another.

After 30 years we have a fair idea of the strengths and limitations of treatment for high blood pressure – but it has taken that long. Remarkably, during that time 'current wisdom' was often – even usually – proved wrong by the results of these controlled trials. Among beliefs held strongly at one time or another were that treating hypertension in the elderly would be dangerous; the young should be treated aggressively; treating very mild hypertension would be valuable; treatment would have a large impact on the risk of coronary disease; diuretics (water tablets) would be dangerous; and β-blockers would prevent coronary complications. These ideas have two things in common: they were all held and defended rigorously at one time, and they were all proved wrong conclusively by large controlled trials. The clear message is that treatment intended for a substantial proportion of the healthy population should not be based on extrapolation from short-term studies or theoretical considerations. It should be based *only* on the results of sound, long-term outcome trials. These lessons must not be forgotten when considering the management of high cholesterol.

High cholesterol and hypertension

High blood cholesterol and high blood pressure have much in common. They are both very common, both are powerful risk factors and, indeed, causes of vascular disease. High cholesterol predisposes particularly to coronary heart disease, and high blood pressure causes stroke and heart failure as well as coronary disease. Both are clinically 'silent', meaning that they cause no symptoms, and therefore have to be detected by some form of screening. Finally, both can be modified either by changing diet or by drug treatment.

Our involvement with cholesterol became inevitable when an overlap with hypertension became apparent. High cholesterol and high blood pressure tend to cluster in the population, so that people with high blood pressure are more likely to have high cholesterol than people with normal blood pressure. Furthermore, the presence together of high cholesterol and high blood pressure in an individual has an effect on coronary risk which is more than additive. Again, the drugs used most widely to treat high blood pressure, diuretics and β-blockers, have small effects on blood cholesterol which have been considered potentially harmful.

A situation was reached where guidelines for treating hypertension were virtually directing that blood cholesterol should be measured in all hypertensive patients, and then lowered if it was high. There were, in turn, several published guidelines directing how high blood cholesterol should be lowered.[1–7] In the circumstances we had to examine the evidence on therapeutic interventions to lower blood cholesterol – and did not like what we found one little bit. The problem was not a lack of controlled trials, for there are plenty of them and they are of at least reasonable quality. Rather, the problem has been a failure to interpret these trials correctly, and even – the ultimate sin – to ignore them entirely. We have concluded that guidelines for managing high cholesterol aimed at ordinary doctors in Britain and, indeed, around the world, are not supported by the available scientific evidence and, in fact, are seriously flawed. In a nutshell, there is no form of treatment to lower high blood cholesterol which is effective, feasible, acceptable and safe. The treatments which are advised all fall down on at least one of these cardinal criteria.

The cholesterol problem
Before discussing the treatments available it is important to set out some facts which are not (or should not be) disputed.

- High blood cholesterol is a very common problem in Britain. Levels of cholesterol above 6.5 mmol/l, which are deemed in guidelines to need follow-up and treatment, are present in no less than 40 per cent of the healthy middle-aged population.

- High blood cholesterol is an important risk factor for coronary disease. In men it is also an important predictor of total cardiovascular mortality. In women it carries much less risk, because their overall risk of coronary disease is much smaller than that of men.

- The risk of high blood cholesterol is multiplied when other major risk factors are also present – particularly high blood pressure and cigarette smoking.

- If we did have an acceptable treatment which lowered blood cholesterol safely, it would undoubtedly prevent coronary heart disease. There is some debate about the magnitude of this effect, but for every one per cent fall in blood cholesterol, coronary events would be reduced by between one and three per cent.[8] Thus a 10 per cent reduction in cholesterol would lower coronary risk by 10–30 per cent, an effect which would undoubtedly be worthwhile.

Guidelines for screening and treating cholesterol

To appreciate the problems with treatment, some knowledge is needed of the guidelines published by various specialist groups,[9] aimed at general practitioners and others such as general physicians or cardiologists. These have been fairly uniform in their recommendations which are summarised below.

- Blood cholesterol should be measured routinely in adults. The minimum recommendation is screening of those at 'high risk', meaning those with other risk factors such as high blood pressure, diabetes or a bad family history. However most guidelines recommend that ideally *all* adults should be screened.

- Those with blood cholesterol above 6.5 mmol/l (40 per cent of the middle-aged population of Britain) should have 'clinical care', meaning they should be given advice to lower cholesterol and followed-up. One should note in passing that doctors who do this are taking on a massive task.

- Diet is the cornerstone of treatment. The 'step 1' or 'general lipid-lowering' diet, discussed below, is the diet advised. This diet is said to lower cholesterol by 10–25 per cent, with estimates varying within this range in different guidelines.

- Most 'patients' will have their cholesterol adequately controlled by this diet. The target blood cholesterol has usually been set at 5.2 mmol/l, but in some guidelines at 5.7 mmol/l. It should be noted that to get from 6.5 mmol/l or higher to these targets requires *minimum* cholesterol falls of 20 per cent or 13 per cent respectively.

- Drugs to lower cholesterol should be considered only when

diet fails, and because of the perceived effectiveness of diet will be needed 'uncommonly' or 'rarely'.

Before leaving these guidelines to consider the evidence, the 'knock-on' effect if diet does not work should be noted. Quite simply 'patients' will either be left with a high blood cholesterol, and the knowledge of it, or will need treatment with cholesterol-lowering drugs. The policy for screening and treatment will be successful only if the diet lowers blood cholesterol by 10–25 per cent, as the guidelines suggest.

The step 1 or general lipid-lowering diet
This diet entails:

- calorie restriction to reduce weight to the ideal

- reduction in total dietary fat to 30 per cent of calories, compared to 40 per cent in the average British diet

- reduction in saturated fats and increase in polyunsaturated fats to achieve a ratio of 1.0

- reduction of cholesterol to 300 mg daily.

In some earlier guidelines more rigorous dietary change (the step 2 diet) was recommended if the step 1 diet did not achieve its aim. This required a further increase in the ratio of saturated:polyunsaturated fats and further reduction in dietary cholesterol, but with total dietary fats still held at 30 per cent of calories. The most recent guidelines have all recommended only the step 1 diet.

The guidelines cite evidence to support a 10–25 per cent reduction in blood cholesterol by this diet, quoting short-term feeding experiments in healthy subjects, uncontrolled trials (which are not reliable), and even trials of much more rigorous dietary fat reduction (which are indeed effective in lowering cholesterol, as discussed later, but were abandoned because they were neither feasible nor palatable). *Not* cited in any of the guidelines are long-term controlled trials, and one might think there were none. In fact there are several discussed below and they are with the question in mind – does the diet work, does it indeed lower cholesterol by 10–25 per cent as is suggested?

Controlled trials of step 1 diet

We have sought out, reviewed and published[10] the results of *all* controlled trials of the step 1 diet of six months or longer (see *Table 1*). The studies identified were performed in eight countries and involved over 10,000 high risk people, all of whom had their blood cholesterol measured, were given appropriate dietary advice by dieticians or doctors, and were followed up. Almost all of those studied were men, a point of considerable importance as there is evidence that women respond less well to diet than men. Some of the people studied had survived a heart attack, some had high blood pressure, and others were selected because they had multiple risk factors for coronary disease. All of them had high blood cholesterol. It is important to note that these trials were performed with expectations that the diet was effective, not that it was ineffective.

To our astonishment the average reduction of blood cholesterol in these trials was not the 10–25 per cent suggested – it was in fact a cholesterol fall of only two per cent, with a range in different trials between zero and four per cent. In only one of these trials was the fall in blood cholesterol (of two per cent) statistically significant. A fall in blood cholesterol of this magnitude will have a negligible impact on coronary risk, and has very little chance of 'controlling' cholesterol in a subject with an initial level of 6.5 mmol/l or higher, as will be discussed below.

The very small cholesterol responses to diet in these trials have been rationalised away on various grounds, none of which are scientifically defensible. The trials are easily large enough to be certain that a real response which is much bigger

Table 1. Controlled trials of Step 1 or equivalent diet to lower cholesterol.

Trial	Setting & subjects*	n	% Men	Duration (years)	Baseline cholesterol (mmol/l)	Change in cholesterol
INTERVENTION ON INDIVIDUAL PATIENTS						
UKHDPP	Factories, high risk	1278	100	5–6	6.6	−0.9%
WHO Euro	Factories, high risk	1898	100	4	6.7	−4.0%
MRFIT[10]	Employees, high risk	6428	100	6	6.2	−2.0%
DART	Hospital, post-MI	982	100	2	6.5	−3.5%
Curzio et al.	Hospital, high risk	61	44	0.5	7.1	0.0%
POPULATION INTERVENTION						
North Karelia	Population	2535	49	10	7.1	−2.0%
Stanford	Population (cohort)	490	47	5.5	5.5	−0.6%
	Population (cross-section)	–	–	5.5	5.4	−1.7%
COMBINED INDIVIDUAL + POPULATION INTERVENTION						
UKHDPP	Factories, all subjects	5373	100	5–6	5.6	+1.0%
WHO Euro	Factories, all subjects	824	100	4	5.6	−2.1%
Goteborg	Male population	1473	100	10	6.5	−0.2%

* abbreviations; MI = myocardial infarction

has not been missed by chance. It has been suggested that control groups (ie, those not given diet advice) may have altered their diets also, thus 'contaminating' the studies and 'diluting' any effect of diet. This is easily checked by looking at absolute changes in cholesterol from baseline values, ignoring the control groups. The cholesterol changes were still very small.[11] It has been suggested that intervention efforts or methods in these trials were inadequate. In the largest trial, the Multiple Risk Factor Intervention Trial in the United States, men and their spouses had 10 weekly group sessions, followed by individual sessions, supervised by a team which included a physician, dieticians, health counsellors and a behavioural psychologist. The diet was intensified during the trial yet, despite all this, the blood cholesterol fell by only two per cent after six years.[12] This is an intensity of intervention effort to which ordinary doctors in this country could not even aspire. It has been suggested that the subjects in these trials were non-compliant with diet but surely, when over 10,000 people in eight different countries are 'non-compliant', the finger has to be pointed at the diet, not at recipients of the advice.

When faced with this evidence there are some who say that these clinical trials are not representative of real life, and that they can 'do better' in ordinary practice. This is the final refuge of those who really have nowhere to hide – 'if science does not support what I believe, I do not believe in science'. There is no way that results in ordinary practice will be better than those in the controlled trials, indeed the opposite is likely to be true. The simple truth is that the diet recommended in all the guidelines is insufficiently intensive to lower cholesterol significantly.

Why has this large body of scientific evidence been ignored by the many experts who have drawn up and published guidelines for management of cholesterol? The charitable explanation is that they simply overlooked the evidence and accepted without question that the diet would lower cholesterol. However this cannot explain the deafening silence which has prevailed since our overview of this evidence was published in the *British Medical Journal*.[13] Furthermore it is impossible to be charitable to new guidelines published since then which *still* state that the step 1 diet lowers cholesterol by 10–25 per cent.[14]

Implications for treatment

The very small response to the step 1 diet destroys the foundation of the management guidelines. The chance of an individual with cholesterol higher than 6.5 mmol/l achieving the target level with this diet is very small. Only one in 25 people will reach even a level of 5.7 mmol/l with the diet, and the chance of reaching the more ambitious target cholesterol of 5.2 mmol/l is remote. The step 1 diet is feasible, acceptable and probably perfectly safe – but it is ineffective. If cholesterol is to be lowered, therefore, we have to consider the alternative treatments available. These are either more rigorous low-fat diets or cholesterol-lowering drugs.

Rigorous dietary fat reduction

Changes in diet *can* lower blood cholesterol substantially and can also reduce the incidence of coronary disease, probably without any adverse effect. However, the controlled trials showing this have all employed dietary fat reduction to levels below 30 per cent – as low as 20 per cent – with increases in the polyunsaturated : saturated ratio to as high as 1.4, and reduction of dietary cholesterol to as little as 150 mg daily. These diets lower blood cholesterol by an average of 13 per cent which would certainly be worthwhile in coronary prevention. However, many of these trials were conducted in captive populations, for example in long-stay institutions (see *Table 2*), and in most of the others the diets were abandoned as unpalatable. In some published reports these diets have been presented as simple and well-accepted, but it is clear that the subjects were very highly selected, and that supervision was extremely intensive to the extent that even special foodstuffs were provided. There is no way that this type of diet could be implemented in ordinary practice with resources available in

Table 2. Controlled trials of very intensive diets to lower cholesterol.

Trial	Setting & subjects	n	% Men	Duration (years)	Baseline cholesterol (mmol/l)	Change in cholesterol
FREE-LIVING SUBJECTS						
Oslo study	Population, high risk	604	100	5	8.3	−13.0%
Leren	Hospital, post-MI	206	100	5	7.7	−13.9%
MRC committee (soya-bean oil)	Hospital, post-MI	169	100	2	7.1	−15.1%
Research committee (low-fat diet)	Hospital, post-MI	81	100	2	6.8	−8.1%
Rose et al. (corn oil)	Hospital, IHD	13	–	2	6.8	−6.5%
INSTITUTIONALISED SUBJECTS						
Minnesota	Mental hospitals	4541	48	1	5.4	−13.5%
Finnish MHS	Mental hospitals	300	100	4.5	7.0	−15.5%
Dayton et al.	Veterans center	163	100	2	6.1	−12.8%

* abbreviations; MI = myocardial infarction;
IHD = ischaemic heart disease

this country at present. These diets *might* be acceptable to individual subjects at extremely high risk of coronary heart disease, for example those who had already suffered a heart attack, but they are likely to be totally unacceptable to the 40 per cent of healthy middle-aged members of our population with cholesterols higher than 6.5 mmol/l. The effect of such diets on the quality of life would also need to be carefully considered. This form of diet intervention is therefore effective and is probably safe but it is not feasible and most unlikely to be acceptable.

Cholesterol-lowering drugs

If the simple step 1 diet is ineffective, and the rigorous low-fat diets unacceptable, cholesterol-lowering drugs will have to be used widely if we are to 'control' high blood cholesterol levels. What is known about these drugs? There have been many controlled trials examining their effect on blood cholesterol, coronary disease, and total deaths. Viewed as a whole, these trials show that drug treatment does lower blood cholesterol and does reduce non-fatal coronary attacks.[15] However total mortality has not been reduced and, indeed, has increased slightly. The worrying observation is that *non-coronary* mortality has been increased substantially and significantly by this form of treatment.[16] It appears that the beneficial effect of these drugs on coronary disease has been balanced and even outweighed by some adverse effect of the treatment.[17] Since these trials were conducted, new cholesterol-lowering drugs have become available, but these have not yet been tested in outcome trials of this kind. The dilemma we face now is whether these drugs will eventually be proved safe, or whether they will also cause the adverse effect on non-coronary mortality observed with the older drugs. This question can be answered only by large long-term trials, and unfortunately it is likely to be some years before we know the answer.

What should be done in the meantime? Opinions differ, with some assuming that the newer cholesterol-lowering drugs are safe until proven otherwise, and therefore willing to prescribe them without apparent misgivings. In our view it is quite wrong to sanction the wide use of these drugs in healthy people who are at relatively low risk of coronary disease until they are *proven* to be safe in the long term. Their use *might* be defended in a small minority of people at extremely high risk of coronary disease, namely those who already have coronary disease and those with the uncommon form of very high cholesterol which runs in families. However, even in these patients the balance of benefit and risk is not clearly established. If it is assumed that the benefit does exceed risk in these patients, it is still neither necessary nor justifiable to screen the whole adult population to identify this very small group at extremely high risk.

Implications for cholesterol screening
Routine cholesterol tests will reveal levels higher than 6.5 mmol/l in 40 per cent of middle-aged Britons, but at present they cannot be offered treatment which is effective, acceptable and safe. Knowing that their cholesterol is unacceptably high, they face the unenviable choice between an ineffective diet, an effective but unpalatable diet, or drug therapy which to date has proved unsafe. This being so, what other arguments are there for having blood cholesterol screened at all? It is suggested that knowledge of blood cholesterol helps predict overall coronary risk, so that *other* measures to reduce risk can be targeted more accurately. However, measurement of cholesterol adds very little to prediction of overall coronary risk using simpler factors such as age, male sex, blood pressure, smoking habit, family history, and the presence of symptoms of coronary disease.[18] It has also been suggested that knowing their cholesterol level may motivate people to modify other coronary risk factors, such as cigarette smoking. However this has been proved not to be so in controlled trials.[19] There is therefore no logical case for widespread cholesterol screening at the present time although measurement of cholesterol *might* be justifiable in patients who already have coronary disease or other forms of artery disease, and also in those with grounds for suspecting the uncommon form of severe familial high cholesterol.

It is significant that even doctors in the United States, the front-running 'know your number' nation, are having second thoughts about cholesterol screening. Recently an editorial in *Circulation*, a prestigious American journal, concluded:

> The new evidence on non-coronary causes of death makes it clear that we should draw back from universal screening and treatment of blood cholesterol for primary prevention in adults. This change in direction – limiting cholesterol screening and intervention to the minority in our population for which the benefits clearly predominate over the harms (those with coronary disease or other reasons for being at comparable very high risk of coronary death) – will not be easy. We need now to pull back our national policies directed at identifying and treating high blood cholesterol in the primary prevention setting and put on hold well-meant desires to intervene while we await convincing evidence that the net effects will be beneficial.[20]

When such serious misgivings are being expressed on the other side of the Atlantic, healthy members of our population should think very carefully before agreeing to a cholesterol test – they are likely to find themselves with a big problem that has no easy solution.

Implications for coronary prevention

There is a widely-held misconception that those like us who argue that the available evidence does not support cholesterol screening and treatment are nihilistic towards coronary prevention. In our case we spend much of our time treating and researching hypertension – with the specific goal of preventing cardiovascular complications, including coronary disease. In fact cholesterol is only one of many factors which contribute to coronary risk, and the conclusion that cholesterol screening is unjustifiable is in no way a recipe for nihilism. For example, strenuous efforts need to be directed towards reducing cigarette smoking which, if successful, would have a major impact on coronary incidence. It is also clear now that treatment of hypertension reduces coronary risk, and healthy adults should have their blood pressure measured as a matter of routine at least every five years. If sustained high blood pressure is detected it should be treated appropriately. A case can also be made for regular exercise appropriate to age and general fitness, and for reducing body weight to the ideal by calorie restriction. Those at very high risk of coronary disease can benefit too from simple treatment with a low daily dose of aspirin, provided they have no contraindication to such treatment.

Rejection of cholesterol screening and treatment on the present evidence has nothing to do with nihilism – it is based on rational therapeutic principles. If in future an acceptable diet is devised which does lower cholesterol effectively, or the newer cholesterol-lowering drugs are proved safe, cholesterol reduction may well win an important role in coronary prevention.

Population intervention to reduce risk
So far we have considered only invervention in individuals, meaning cholesterol measurement followed by medical treatment, which is very much in the domain of the general practitioner or general physician. An alternative approach is to aim for cholesterol reduction in the whole population, using health education measures through schools, the media, leaflets, etc. There are points in favour of this approach compared to individual intervention. It is more efficient in economic terms; it need not be directed at a single risk factor, such as cholesterol, but can readily include health education on other factors such as smoking, alcohol, being overweight and lack of exercise. Above all, it carries no risk of turning healthy people into patients. Those exposed to health education of this type can choose to follow the advice or ignore it, according to their wishes. The major drawback is that population education

programmes to reduce blood cholesterol by altering diet have not proved effective. No scientifically sound randomised controlled trial of population advice to lower cholesterol has shown a significant reduction in blood cholesterol (see *Table 1*). There has been some decline in dietary fat consumption in this country in recent years, and this may well be beneficial. However, an intensive campaign to reduce population fat intake further is unlikely to prove worthwhile, judging by the outcome of these controlled trials.

Wider implications

Our brief sally into the world of cholesterol has prompted many more general thoughts. The medical profession appears to have a short collective memory and does not learn well from history. Some 20 years ago, clofibrate was widely used throughout the world as routine treatment for high cholesterol because of evidence that it lowered blood cholesterol and, subsequently, that it also prevented non-fatal coronary attacks. However, when put to the test in very large outcome trials, it transpired that clofibrate did more harm than good, because it increased non-coronary deaths substantially and significantly.[21] The evidence for this was so strong that its use was virtually abandoned. The evidence now available to support the use of cholesterol-lowering drugs is remarkably similar to the evidence then available for clofibrate. Furthermore, several of the new cholesterol-lowering drugs now in general use are very close relatives of clofibrate. Those who prescribe these newer drugs without any concern that they too may do more harm than good must be supreme optimists.

In recent times doctors have been bombarded with consensus statements, treatment protocols, management guidelines and the like. Those who draw up such guidelines should bear in mind that they may have a major impact on ordinary practice, and indeed hope to do so. They have a duty to consider meticulously *all* the scientific evidence available, and to avoid at all costs selective use of this evidence. This has evidently not been done when drawing up guidelines for screening and treating cholesterol. We should be grateful for the conservatism of the medical profession in Britain – the fact that most doctors have not acted on these cholesterol guidelines is a blessing.

Finally, it is pleasing to note that the Department of Health seems to have got it absolutely right on this occasion. New initiatives on coronary prevention for general practice target cigarette smoking, detection and treatment of hypertension, obesity, alcohol use, and physical inactivity. A healthy diet is also recommended – but the word cholesterol is conspicuous by its absence from the Department of Health guidelines.

Health of the Nation: a critical appraisal of Government policy on mental health

Frank Holloway

Introduction

The priority for mental health in *Health of the Nation* is 'to reduce ill-health and death caused by mental illness' which is broken down into three 'targets'. First, to improve significantly the health and social functioning of mentally ill people. Secondly, to reduce the overall suicide rate by at least 15 per cent by the year 2000. And, thirdly, to reduce the suicide rate of severely mentally ill people by at least 33 per cent by the year 2000.[1] But are these targets achievable? There is, after all, absolutely no evidence that the onset of serious mental illness can be prevented. The history of psychiatry is littered with frustrated hopes of effective prevention. The Child Guidance movement in Britain,[2] the Community Mental Health Centre movement in the United States,[3] the application of crisis theory to mental health services,[4] and the unfulfilled aspirations of psychotherapeutically-oriented Social Psychiatrists[5] are examples of the failure of previous preventive strategies. Effective prevention must be based on an understanding of the aetiology of mental illness.[6] The handful of successful demonstration projects that have been published, largely targeted towards the role of social support in the prevention of affective disorders, should be seen as a stimulus to further research rather than large-scale service development.[7] Clearly, then, it is necessary to examine more closely the reality of medical services for the mentally ill.

Health of the Nation: its value and limitations – external constraints

Health and welfare policy in Britain is profoundly influenced by factors that are not under the control of the Department of Health, including demographic changes resulting in an ageing population with fewer available carers; the rising costs of medical technology (and social care); the explosion in the costs of social security provision for the residential care of the elderly; and rising expectations of health and welfare services. The result is severe strain on health and social welfare budgets at a time when resources are increasingly limited.

Government strategy

A number of general trends can be identified in the Government response to difficult health and social welfare issues of which the overwhelming priority is to contain expenditure. There is a consistent move away from universal provision towards approaches that target 'those most in need'. Allied to which is a move away from budgets that are not cash-limited (notably mainstream social security) towards cash limits (for example the institution of the social fund and the transfer of responsibility for funding residential care to local authorities). Lip-service is paid to the maximum devolution of responsibility: in reality this often means 'devolution of debt' as the centre is protected from the odium attached to difficult decisions. At the same time, paradoxically, there is a trend towards increasing central control, particularly at the expense of local authorities.

The contracting out of services is another characteristic feature of policy, with reliance placed on the marketplace as a mechanism for encouraging the efficiency of services whilst maintaining quality. Contracting out implies casualisation of the labour force, with the introduction of short-term contracts and a freer market in labour.

The theory of preventing mental illness

There are a number of initiatives aimed at achieving *Health of the Nation*'s mental health targets. These include measures to improve 'information and understanding', the 'development of comprehensive local services' and the 'further development of good practice'.[8] More specifically, a survey to establish national baseline data on the population prevalence of mental illness is promised; provider units are to be required to sample the morbidity of their patients; arrangements for the audit of suicide are to be included in service contracts; and the care programme approach is to be further emphasised. Joint purchasing of local services is to be established, whilst Regional Health Authorities are instructed to ensure that a full programme of mental hospital re-provision is in place. Good practice guidelines are to be developed between primary and secondary care services 'for the assessment and management of common psychiatric conditions'. Within 'secondary care' comprehensive services are to be provided, including 'family intervention services, direct education of users, education and support of carers [and] genetic counselling if requested'. The needs of mentally disordered offenders receive specific mention as does the issue of benzo-diazepine abuse.

Making prevention work

It is clearly hoped that, with further research, the first mental health target ('to improve significantly the health and social functioning of mentally ill people') will be adequately implemented. But, in the absence of a clear goal for mental health services within *Health of the Nation*, there is a danger that the rhetoric of change will suffice. Currently, throughout Britain, service contracts, quality standards, business plans, mission statements and community care plans are being churned out by health and social care purchasers and providers, which at times seem to relate poorly to the reality of service provision.

One possible way of assessing the achievability of the *Health of the Nation* targets, ill-defined as they are, is to set out some key features of good mental illness services that would be generally agreed by interested parties to be of significant importance to the welfare of people with a severe mental illness. The probable impact of current policy on these key service attributes may then be systematically reviewed.

The possible impact of policy on the welfare of the mentally ill

It is generally agreed that mental health services should be comprehensive, local and integrated.[9] But many factors in current policy, the purchaser/provider split, the health/social care divide, the hospital/community distinction and incipient competition between providers for service contracts all make the vision of a seamless service spanning agencies and locations seem improbable.

In theory, 'care management' is to be the glue that will bind the efforts of community care providers into a coherent 'package of care' tailored to the individual. Unfortunately no-one is quite clear what care management means in terms of practical services to those with mental illness who seek 'social care'.

Targeting of services to those most in need is a sensible response to restricted resources but, again, it is unclear whether GP fund-holders will be happy to purchase expensive community services for people with a long-term mental illness. Many may choose to purchase psychology, counselling and community psychiatric nursing services for more vocal patients presenting with psycho-social crises and neurotic disorders. Similarly, there must be concern over the commitment of social service departments to the community care of people with a mental illness, whose needs have to be balanced against more immediate political priorities such as the elderly and people with a mental handicap.[10]

Moreover, the purchaser/provider split encourages 'providers' to market their wares, concentrating on what can be sold in favour of alternative and less marketable solutions to patients' problems. The result of the recent reforms may be paradoxically to increase reliance on residential and hospital care. For example, the logic of current policy is for purchasers of health care to constrain providers to retreat to a 'core business' that does not include long-term supportive day care and sheltered work, despite evidence for its efficacy.[11] The ability of local authorities to sustain a comprehensive range of mental illness day care services, given their previous lack of commitment to the area, and their future dire financial situation, must be in serious doubt.

Mental health services should provide a rapid and effective response to crises. Although there is evidence that a proportion of actually ill patients presenting for admission can be successfully managed by community teams or acute day care[12] the recurrent bed crisis in London is severely undermining the capacity of clinicians to respond appropriately to requests for admission.[13] The situation may well be exacerbated by the full implementation of 'Caring for People' which is likely to curtail the discharge of patients into supported residential accommodation.[14]

Finally, a crucial element of a good quality service for the mentally ill is the need for long-term individual support from an experienced professional. Skilled help can enable patients to regain a sense of self despite continuing psychotic symptoms,[15] or provide a degree of support until adventitious life experiences precipitate positive change.[16] The role of the 'care manager' precludes an individual relationship with the client.[17] If the role of health care professionals is to be restricted to the reduction of symptoms, which may be construed as the prescription of antipsychotic medication, personal supportive care may disappear.

The suicide targets

Health of the Nation identifies suicide as a major public health problem. There are ambitious targets for the reduction of the overall suicide rate and of the suicide rate amongst people in contact with psychiatric services. Coroners differ dramatically in their tendency to come to a verdict of suicide[18] and to counteract this effect the *Health of the Nation* targets include undetermined deaths. Two initiatives are proposed to achieve the target reduction: first, a programme of training primary care and mental health professionals in the recognition and management of depression and suicidal behaviour; secondly, an audit of suicides by patients in contact with services.

Model training programmes have been developed that appear to be able to influence the knowledge and attitudes of GPs.[19] The British Confidential Inquiry[20] identified potentially remediable factors in a significant proportion of suicides in contact with the local services, notably failure to recognise the degree of suicide risk, absence without leave from the inpatient ward and a conflictual relationship between caring staff and the patients (who were frequently identified as manipulative or demanding). Other studies have linked suicide to exit events, including leaving hospital. In some areas pressure on beds has led to the accelerated discharge of patients who may not be clinically well. As the level of morbidity in inner-city inpatient units rises, the ward environment may become intolerable for patients with depression[21] and absconding can become a regular feature of ward life. It is possible that current trends in psychiatric practice may actually increase the risk of suicide amongst patients in contact with services.

There is absolutely no evidence that the sensible initiatives described above will have a substantial effect on suicide rates. Education of GPs, however effective, is surely unlikely to bring about suicide-preventing change in the one in 30,000 consultations that a GP will have in the five years before a patient on his list consults and then goes on to kill himself. Moreover, policy fails to acknowledge the impact of the broader, largely unexplained, factors that influence suicide rates over time and between cultures.   ⊚

Conclusion

Health of the Nation is a well-intentioned document. The broad aim of mental health policy (reducing psychiatric disability) is admirable, if inadequately thought out. One danger of this lack of clarity is the substitution of less appropriate aims for a mental health policy. It is therefore not surprising that the Mental Health Task Force has interpreted *Health of the Nation* in terms of what might be described as systems-level goals. Their work programme comprises:

- *a service modernisation programme* to ensure that each regional health authority has a plan to close the remaining long-stay institutions by the end of the century

- *a market intelligence programme* to provide an information database on mental illness services and to offer managers information on the options available in moving from long-stay institutional care

- *a customer satisfaction programme* to make recommendations on achieving the involvement of patients and their carers in the development of services

- *a programme to promote public understanding* of the policy of care in the community for mentally ill people.

These programmes have little obvious relationship to the welfare of mentally ill people and a lot to do with forcing through pre-existing Government policy.

Health of the Nation sets out a number of welcome initiatives for mental health services, which include the development of good practice guidelines, encouragement for the continuing education and training of mental health practitioners and the development of simple and reliable measures for the assessment of the outcome of psychiatric care. The NHS Research and Development strategy is to focus on the priorities set out in *Health of the Nation* which will hopefully catalyze research into the provision of mental health services. However, it is doubtful that any positive effects from these initiatives will outweigh the generally negative impact of current Government policy on the welfare of people with a severe mental illness.

8

Does health education work?

James Le Fanu

Introduction

Health education is an unexciting subject of marginal intellectual content. In essence, and this is certainly the overriding public impression, it takes the form of advertising slogans – or rather admonitions – which, were they complied with, are presumed to improve the health of the nation: don't drink and drive; wear a condom; smoking kills; eat healthily, etc.

There is, of course, slightly more to health education than this. Both the BBC and commercial television have made a point in recent years of broadcasting series with a strong health education input which substantiate and attempt to justify these slogans, especially those concerned with healthy eating. Nurses in general practice and, to a less extent GPs themselves, make the point of getting a spot of 'health education' into their consultations and it is also a modest part of the school curriculum.

On these intellectually modest foundations, however, rests much of the Government's strategy for improving the Health of the Nation, laid out in the document of that title published in July 1992. Major initiatives to reduce the toll from coronary heart disease and stroke, from cancers of the stomach and lung, sexually transmitted diseases and accidents in both the young and old are to be achieved by modifying, through health education, those aspects of human behaviour – particularly food, sexual and smoking hazards – which are allegedly responsible for them.

89

It is therefore of some interest, with the Government's policies so firmly focused on these eminently desirable targets, to inquire whether health education works. That is to say, whether it has a chance of preventing in some large measure these serious problems.

Alternative perceptions of health education

A cursory examination of the literature reveals two apparently contradictory findings. First, scientific attempts to evaluate health education programmes almost all show that it is actually very difficult to get people to change their behaviour by cajoling them to do so. On the other hand, certain spectacular achievements in public health in recent years, notably the precipitous decline of almost 50 per cent in premature death from coronary heart disease in the United States and the fact that there has been no heterosexual AIDS epidemic in this country, have been consistently claimed as evidence of the great triumph of health education in persuading people to change their lifestyles.

It is, of course, important to know which of these two perceptions of the value of health education is correct because they certainly cannot both be. If it is the former, then the targets in the Government's health policy are a mirage and attempts to achieve them a waste of resources. If the latter, then it could be argued that so manifestly potent is health education that it deserves much more than the current 0.5 per cent of the total NHS budget.

There are other reasons why it is important to know the answer. The effectiveness or otherwise of health education programmes in changing behaviour and therefore patterns of disease is in itself an important experimental test of the sometimes contentious hypotheses of the causation of these diseases. While none would dispute that smoking causes lung cancer, some are sceptical about the role of fat consumption in heart disease or stroke. If changing patterns of food consumption really have produced major changes in the pattern of disease, this is important experimental evidence for this contention. If, however, the incidence of heart disease has fallen while fat consumption has remained virtually unchanged, this is strong experimental evidence against the theory and, indeed, of the whole strategy that seeks to influence patterns of disease by encouraging people to make major changes in their diet.

Secondly, health education like any other branch of medicine is not without its 'side effects' which would be – as with the case of drugs – acceptable if it worked, but unacceptable if it does not. These side effects would include frightening the public with misleading concepts about the risk of everyday life, the linking of pleasurable activities like eating and sex with disability and death. Do fish and chips clog up the arteries? Is unprotected casual heterosexual intercourse very risky? For those unfortunate enough to suffer from coronary heart disease or stroke, the health education message might have the 'side effect' of blaming the victim where the sufferers believe that their misfortune is in large measure their own fault.

Then the health education message must by definition simplify and highlight issues. This may be acceptable if they have the desired effect, but if they do not then perhaps the only result is to give the public a false understanding of the nature of disease and an inappropriate sense of doom. Lastly, we need to know if health education works for important political reasons. Over the last decade the Conservative Government has enormously increased its direct involvement in the private lives of the nation through its resourcing of health education programmes. There are two sound reasons for regretting this development: it reinforces the ethos of the nanny state in which the notion that individuals are responsible for their own lives is marginalised; further, and this particularly applies to the AIDS campaign, it has been argued by, for example, the Chief Rabbi, the campaigns appear to endorse a moral message which sanctions casual sexual intercourse as long as it is performed 'safely'. To this extent health education can be said to have influenced the moral tone of the nation.

What should be the aim of health education?

Before examining the specific question of whether health education works, it is useful to meditate on the task it has set out to achieve. The goal of health education, according to Green, is to 'obtain individual and voluntary health acts'.[1] This makes it qualitatively different from most other forms of education whose aim is to impart knowledge or intellectual skills. It is not enough simply to educate the public about, say, the dangers of saturated fat, health education has to go further and actually get people to act on that knowledge.

This, self-evidently, is unlikely to be easy especially when, as is widely assumed, those whose health behaviour perhaps needs changing most may well be just those who are least susceptible to health education messages. Further, the nature of the behaviour change that is sought is frequently, as in the case of smoking, alcohol, food and sex, pleasurable, not to say 'addictive' and part of a wider cultural pattern of behaviour within social groups. It is thus clearly not readily amenable to change just from the knowledge that such practices might be harmful.

This is made clear by appreciating the gap between *knowledge* and *practice*. Many, indeed in Britain virtually everyone, knows and believes that smoking is harmful but this by itself clearly does not prevent up to a third of the adult population from practising the habit. The bridge between knowledge and action (or behavioural change), is *intention*, so the central task of health education must be to influence that intention.[2] This requires some form of social engineering to change the cultural climate in such a way that everyone sees the desired need for change and then by, for example, breaking that change down into small steps, makes it more easily achievable.

There is, however, a wider dimension to this issue which must also be appreciated. Mass media campaigns are generally accepted to be ineffective. Leventhal calculates their positive effect to be around 10 per cent,[3] but spread over a long period of time, like a decade, they can influence the cultural perception of the risk, of smoking for example, in a way that makes it socially highly desirable to stop. When the decision to quit is made, then the central issue becomes one of individual willpower, in which 'health education' probably has little or nothing to contribute, though the help or support of health professionals like doctors in giving encouragement may well be helpful. Thus, viewed in the short term, health education may seem to be ineffective, but in the long term it can have considerable 'hidden benefits'.

Assessments of health education's effectiveness

With these thoughts in mind it is appropriate to return to the specific evidence of the effectiveness of health education which has been comprehensively reviewed by Dr Alex Gatherer and others in their publication, *Is Health Education Effective?* published by the Health Education Council,[4] (the very body which under this title and the later, Health Education Authority, has been responsible for so many campaigns). In general, Dr Gatherer points out

A majority of the reported studies appeared to be inadequately planned and their findings too confused, vague and insufficiently controlled to be of much educational or practical value to those who may wish to put the findings into practice. The educational projects show a great deal of repetition, the same concepts being studied and the same type of results being obtained over and over again.

The review covers several aspects of health education but I will restrict most of my comments to the mass media campaigns as these are much the most significant and expensive, and are probably the only realistic method of reaching the adult population en masse.

The 49 relevant studies are examined in terms of their measurable influence on knowledge, attitude change and behavioural change. Only three of the studies attempt to measure the degree of increase in knowledge and, where they do, the figure is a modest six per cent. This is not necessarily surprising as the knowledge-generating potential of these campaigns is circumscribed because most people already know that, for example, it is dangerous to drink and drive, or smoking is harmful, though they are entitled to be slightly confused about the precise nature of a 'healthy diet'.

Still, the results cited are discouraging. A five-year cancer education study in Canada from 1958 found 'little or no general increase in knowledge and the subjects in the experimental area know no more about cancer symptoms than the controlled area'.[5] Another campaign on tar yields in cigarettes showed an increase in knowledge over a two-year period from eight per cent to 27 per cent – but this did not influence the number smoking milder cigarettes.[6]

Changes in 'attitude' are evident where smoking is concerned, though again the effect is modest because of the virtually universal assumption that smoking is harmful anyhow. In one study over a five-year period between 1970 and 1975, the percentage of those who thought that smoking was harmful to health increased from 87 to 90 per cent.[7]

In several instances however, as the review acknowledges, the attitudinal change following a health campaign 'is in the opposite direction of that desired'. An anti-alcohol campaign in Tyne and Tees in 1975 was followed by an increase in the frequency and quantity of teenage alcohol consumption.[8] This phenomenon seems to be a particular problem for drug campaigns. When the film 'The Man with the Golden Arm' starring Frank Sinatra and Kim Novak, which dealt with the hero's fight against addiction was widely shown in the United States in the early 1970s, the general verdict of addicts who saw the film was that it 'legitimised' addiction. None stopped taking drugs.[9]

The critical question, of course, is whether health education actually changes behaviour. Here the review comments:

> Short term changes of behaviour tended to disappear after a few months; if continued throughout the year, the long term effect is no greater than a 10 per cent change. Repeated campaigns may show a positive result for the first or second exposure, but little improvement or even a regression subsequently.

Thus, an evaluation of the Health Education Council's anti-smoking in pregnancy campaign,[10] the Scottish Health Education Council's 1970 campaign on alcoholism,[11] the HEC's 1972 anti-smoking campaign[12] and the 1977 Cancer Week in New Zealand on breast self-examination were all quite clearly ineffective.[13]

Can health education be made more effective?
If good results are to be obtained it seems to be necessary to combine mass media campaigns with much more intensive health education techniques as is shown by the North Karelia Project[14] and the Stamford Three County Study.[15] Both of these involved a concerted effort to supplement the mass media campaigns with specialised training of health personnel, the promotion of healthy food in shops and, in addition, a random section of the population were interviewed, examined

and exalted to change their lifestyle. In the North Karelia Study there was a highly significant reduction in risk factor behaviour for coronary heart disease after five years, and in the Stamford study an especially targeted high risk group had reduced their risk factor behaviour by almost 30 per cent after two years. Essentially this means there had been major changes in smoking and exercise habit and moves towards a more 'healthy diet'.

This sort of *blitzkrieg* approach to health education obviously can work, but as Dr John Farquhar who organised the Stamford project comments, the resources required are so enormous as to make this method of approach generally inapplicable. Further, though both programmes achieved important changes in those of aspects of lifestyle to which coronary heart disease is attributed, in neither was there a significant decline in actual coronary heart disease mortality compared to controlled areas.

Concluding this overview of the mass media campaigns, Dr Gatherer and his colleagues comment

> There is a common assumption that the mass media have a powerful influence on our lives, but these evaluation studies have shown their effect is not very great, especially upon the individual.

However, they leave open the possibility already mentioned that

> The long term effect over decades of media campaigns in helping to bring about a gradual change in the climate of opinion, and thus in the definition of acceptable behaviour, should not be underrated.

This, I am sure, is fair comment, certainly in relation to smoking. Thus the famous 1962 Royal College of Physicians report on smoking and health accelerated the decline in cigarette smoking from 4.6 to 9 per cent that year, and the publicity generated by the 1965 ban on television advertising of cigarettes had a similar effect. The scale of decline faded in time, but the cumulative effect of anti-smoking propaganda over two decades has been associated with a major decline in smoking from 52 to 33 per cent of the population.

As Dr Warner has pointed out, the true effect is certainly much greater than this because the campaigns have stopped in its tracks an incremental increase in per capita cigarette smoking from 1953 onwards which, had it continued, would by 1975 have reached 5,400 per year when, in fact, the figure is just over 4,000 as shown in *Figure 1*.[16] Dr Warner comments,

> This analysis suggests that per capita consumption would have been from one fifth to one third larger than it actually is, had the years of anti-smoking publicity never materialised.

More recent developments, particularly the passive smoking campaign with the voluntary smoking ban in places of work that has come in its wake, are likely to accelerate considerably the fall in the number of smokers. Thus, much of the credit for this almost universal acceptance of 'this is the way to go' must go to the relentless anti-smoking campaigns for having prepared the way.

Are health educationists' claims of success always valid?

It is important, however, to know whether smoking is a typical example of what health education can achieve or whether it is exceptional. Here we come to the second requirement in evaluating the effectiveness of health education. The studies that have been considered do not in a general way support the contention of that effectiveness. On the other hand, the belief that health education is of value persists because of its

supposed spectacular achievement in producing a major decline in coronary heart disease in the last two decades, particularly in the United States, and, to a lesser extent, in
containing the AIDS epidemic.

It is difficult to reconcile the two sources of evidence of
relative lack of success and spectacular success so it is important to try to assess whether these instances are correctly
attributed to the effects of health education or simply myths
perpetuated by those in the health education business to keep
themselves in work.

Figure 1. Actual and predicted per capita cigarette
consumption, 1947–1974

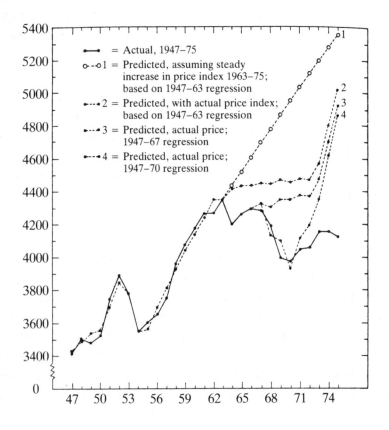

The one central assumption which sustains the credibility of the potent value of preventive medicine generally, and health education in particular, is that the precipitous decline of coronary heart disease in the United States has been brought about by the widespread adoption of a healthy lifestyle: the fall in cigarette consumption, a change to a 'healthier diet' and increased exercise have together, it is argued, brought about a fall in CHD mortality of over 50 per cent.

Thus the well-known NACNE Report, which has become the bible of health educationists to justify their campaign in favour of fat reduction in the diet, makes the following observation:

> Compared with other Western nations Britain has a poor record in the prevention of CHD, the rates in recent years showing only a very slight decline compared to those in the USA.[17]

However, the attribution of the decline of coronary heart disease to a healthy lifestyle might be an example of the '*post hoc, ergo propter-hoc*' fallacy where, because the decline in coronary heart disease appears to coincide with changes to a healthy lifestyle, so coronary heart disease must be caused by an unhealthy lifestyle.

To simplify matters I will just examine four countries, the United States, Canada, New Zealand and Australia, from 1950 until 1988.[18] The details are shown in *Figure 2*. The most striking point already noted is the way in which these mortality trends all run together, which presupposes that in all these different societies, across all generations and classes, there has been a remarkable synchrony of change in social habits.

What about the pattern of food consumption? Before discussing this final crucial piece of data it is necessary to know that dietary changes have to be fairly substantial to influence cholesterol levels and so subsequent risk of coronary heart disease. Thus, the dietary changes promoted in the Mr Fit Trial to reduce fat consumption from 40 to 30 per cent of total

Figure 2. The rise and fall of heart disease 1950–1980 compared with changes in fat consumption

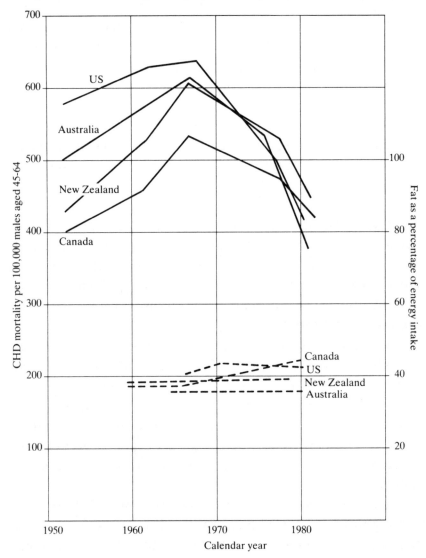

energy intake required the drinking of skimmed milk, abjuring cream, using margarine as a spread, using only low fat cheeses, restricting eggs to one or two a week, avoiding all rich cakes, puddings and pastries and markedly reducing the amount of meat.[19] To begin to explain the changing pattern of coronary heart disease seen in these graphs requires first, that in the 1930s and 1940s fat consumption rose markedly and then in the 1950s and 1960s it fell to an equal degree. This would seem most unlikely to have occurred as patterns of food consumption remain remarkably stable within nations as is evinced by the available data. From the 1950s onwards total fat consumption has remained remarkably static.[20] Certainly there have been small changes in the ratio of polyunsaturated to saturated fats but these are essentially trivial and insufficient to influence substantially the risk of coronary heart disease. It should be pointed out that this lack of parellelism between patterns of coronary heart disease and food consumption applies to virtually every country examined.

It might be that changes in other risk factors like cigarette smoking were important, but the point being made here that the changing pattern of coronary heart disease is attributable to a shift to a healthy diet is clearly unsubstantiated. To emphasise the significance of this point, *Figure 3* shows the striking parallelism between alcohol consumption and liver cirrhosis over time.[21] The contrast to coronary heart disease and fat consumption patterns could not be more marked.

So whatever has caused the decline in coronary heart disease, a shift to a healthy diet does not seem to be one of the reasons. This does not mean that health education may not work in other spheres of life, merely that the claim it is likely to do so because it has proved so efficacious in coronary heart disease is unfounded.

Figure 3. Mortality rate from cirrhosis of the liver in the UK compared to national alcohol consumption

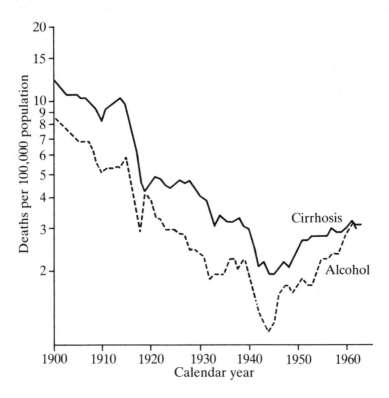

Is health education cost effective?

Finally, I turn to the highest profile of all health education campaigns in recent years – the campaign to control the spread of AIDS. The sums spent between 1986 and 1992 have by any criteria been colossal, totalling a staggering £150 million. The most visible part of this has been the sum of approximately £10 million a year spent on television and billboard campaigns directed, after the initial 'don't die of ignorance' campaign, primarily at the dangers of acquiring the infection by casual heterosexual intercourse. It is possible that the pattern of the AIDS epidemic in this country, with the steady rise from very small numbers in 1983 to a plateau in 1987/88 of just over 1,000 cases a year, and the subsequent modest decline can be attributed in part to these campaigns, but the evidence is not encouraging.

It was apparent from the very earliest days of the AIDS epidemic, long before any substantial funds were allocated to health education, that knowledge of the seriousness of the disease and the possibility that it was transmitted by an infections agent – even though the HIV virus had yet to be identified – resulted in a major change in sexual behaviour amongst homosexuals.

Thus, as early as September 1983, Dr Golubjatnikov of the University of Wisconsin, writing in *The Lancet*, reported a major fall amongst the cohort of homosexuals in the number of 'sexual partners in the previous thirty days' over the preceding year. For example, the numbers reporting '10 or more partners' had fallen from approximately 40 per cent of those interviewed to less than 10 per cent.[22]

There were similar changes in Britain as can be shown by changes in incidence of diseases transmitted in the same way as AIDS, such as rectal gonorrhoea and hepatitis B. *Figure 4* shows the changing incidence of rectal gonorrhoea in male homosexuals in Leicester between 1982 and 1990 and almost exactly the same pattern has been reported in Leeds.[23] Here it must be noted that the major fall occurred from 1983/84 with only a small further decline from 1986 to 1988 when no cases were recorded. However, almost immediately the number of cases started climbing again.

From this it would seem that the significant change in homosexual behaviour had already occurred well before the launch of the high profile health education campaigns of 1986 onwards and perhaps significantly, despite increasing funds allocated year on year, the campaigns failed to prevent an almost immediate relapse into unsafe sexual practices.

The overwhelming thrust of the campaigns has however been directed at preventing HIV transmission through casual heterosexual intercourse by promoting 'safe sex' and condom

Figure 4. Annual frequency of gonorrhoea in homosexuals in Leicester

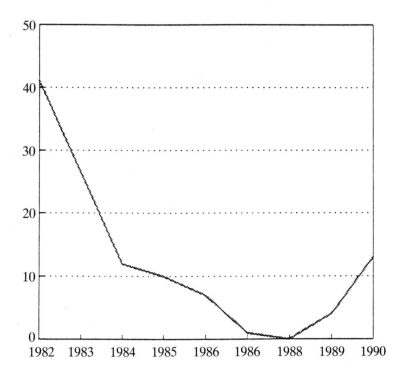

use in particular. It is conceivable that a heterosexual epidemic may have been prevented by this means, though this was never very likely in view of the very low levels of infection amongst heterosexuals who were not in an at risk group (1.2 per cent of the total).[24] In addition, a study of sexual and contraceptive lifestyle of young people to 1992 found that 89 per cent of respondents saw little or no chance of HIV infection in the next few years, with most saying they did not feel the need to bother to use a condom.[25]

In summary, homosexuals had adopted safe sex practices long before the high profile campaign started in 1986 and started relapsing back into unsafe practices from 1988 onwards. The campaign directed towards heterosexuals does not seem to have convinced young people of the putative dangers of HIV transmission and it would thus seem unlikely that the health education campaigns have prevented a heterosexual epidemic. All in all, this seems a rather poor return on an investment of £150 million.

Conclusion

The question 'Does Health Education Work?' will mean different things to different people. To educationists it might mean the health message being understood and assimilated, to a doctor it might mean does it result in a change in 'risky form' of behaviour like smoking or drinking alcohol to excess. However, as part of a public health strategy the bottom line, the criterion of effectiveness, must be can it reduce the incidence of diseases? For only by this criterion can one judge whether the *Health of the Nation* targets for preventive measures can be achieved and whether the resources allocated to health education are justified.

As we have seen – and, indeed, as the HEC's own evaluations show – health education is not effective, the only important success is in reducing smoking and has come about from a protracted campaign waged over many years, while the claims of spectacular success of health education in the reduction of coronary heart disease and control of the AIDS epidemic cannot be substantiated. My answer to the question 'does health education work?' is regrettably, very rarely.

9

The costs of screening

Mark Charny

The different faces of screening

There is considerable confusion over the value of prevention, as it encompasses so many quite different activities, for example preventing heart disease by persuading adults to eat less fat, preventing road accidents with better road layout, phenylketonuria (PKU) with a blood test at birth, or cervical and breast cancer with screening programmes.

Generally any manoeuvre which depends upon changing behaviour through persuasion is more difficult and less likely to succeed than one which does not. As totalitarian politicians have discovered, people are very resilient, and in the end most resist even intense indoctrination of a kind which would be quite unacceptable in Western democracies.

Changing behaviour by altering the environment in which people live works better. Improving road design or changing prices through taxes or subsidies is a more certain way of ensuring that the desired results are obtained. Although the original costs of environmental change are usually much higher than reaching people through individual programmes, the outcome cost may be much lower because the manoeuvre is generally more effective as well as more efficacious.

Finally there are manoeuvres which resemble – socially and technically – the interaction between professionals and patients. Screening for PKU and cervical and breast cancer are examples. Screening, like other preventive measures, is usually considered to be straightforward, 'a good thing'. In this chapter I want to show the philosophical complexity behind screening programmes and the enormous range of cost effectiveness between them.

Screening – the theory

A screening programme requires the application of a particular test in a planned and predetermined way to an identified group of people who do not have symptoms in order to decide whether individuals are more likely to have a disease than would be expected if they were simply picked at random. The purpose of identifying this higher chance of having the disease is to decide who should have a definitive diagnostic test. Thus, a 'suspicious' shadow on a mammogram must be further investigated by a breast biopsy to determine if it is, or is not malignant. These definitive tests are typically more expensive and/or carry more risks, and/or are more uncomfortable than the screening test. This process is shown in *Figure 1*.

Figure 1. The screening process

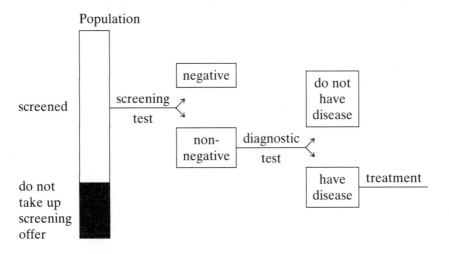

There are four possible outcomes of a screening test (shown in *Table 1*) and, as is clear, the patient benefits in only one of them – a 'true positive'.

Table 1. How a test classifies people

	Actually have disease	Actually do not have disease
Test result abnormal	true positive	false positive
Test result normal	false negative	true negative

In the other three the information derived is either purposeless (true negative) or misleading (false positive/false negative) and those in these categories can be said to be made 'worse off' by screening, as shown in *Table 2*.

Any screening programme must therefore try to make sure that the losses to these three groups are outweighed by the benefit to the first group. Even this may be difficult to define; for instance, for every two terminations of pregnancy which avoid the birth of children who would otherwise be born with spina bifida and survive, it has been estimated that at least one pregnancy is terminated. Is this an acceptable balance between the gains in one situation and losses in another?

Table 2. Gains and losses for the four groups identified in Table 1

	Gains	Losses
True positive	diagnosed earlier, treated earlier, better quantity and/or quality of life	none significant, possible lifetime of taking drug treatment and viewing self as 'ill'
False positive	none	unnecessary worry, may have unnecessary treatment which may be unpleasant or dangerous, cost of screening, further assessment, treatment, etc
True negative	none significant*	time and effort of participating in the programme, cost of screening
False negative	none	false reassurance which may postpone them seeking health care when symptoms appear, cost of screening

* Note that it is often suggested that this group gains by being reassured that they are healthy. This argument is fallacious: the anxiety is engendered by the existence of the screening programme in the first place, and it is illogical to consider as a benefit of a programme the remedy of a harm which the programme has itself caused.

This is clearly a very tricky situation and it should come as no surprise that no less than 10 sound principles have been enumerated that should be fulfilled before a screening programme is undertaken:

• The condition sought should be an important health problem

• There should be an accepted treatment for patients with recognised disease

• Facilities for diagnosis and treatment should be available

• There should be a recognisable latent or early symptomatic stage

- There should be a suitable test or examination

- The test should be acceptable

- The natural history of the disease, including latent to declared disease, should be adequately understood

- There should be an agreed policy on whom to treat as patients

- The cost of case-finding (including diagnosis and treatment of patients diagnosed) should be economically balanced in relation to possible expenditure on medical care as a whole

- There should be an intervention of proven value

To what extent do current screening programmes conform to these basic principles? First, with regards to the suitability of the test or examination, there are three performance characteristics: the ability to discriminate between those with the disease and those without it; the ability to give the same answer from time to time and place to place (reliability); and the relationship to the ultimate objective of the programme (validity). But when screening for cervical cancer, for example, research has repeatedly shown that pathologists reading the same set of smears not only disagree much of the time with each other, but even with themselves! So, while there are some grounds for believing that the cervical cancer programme may reduce mortality from cancer of the cervix, the connection between the test result and the objective of reducing cervical cancer mortality is uncertain, and the reliability of the test is relatively poor.

As to acceptability, if the test is unpleasant people will not cooperate with the programme. In this case the test itself may work (be efficacious) but the failure of clients to cooperate may render the *programme* relatively ineffective. For instance, the test used in screening for blood in faeces in order to detect cancers of the large bowel at an early – and more treatable – stage performs quite well in theory, but many people are understandably reluctant to provide faecal samples, for example, the uptake rate in a trial in Nottingham was only 38 per cent.

Breast cancer provides an illustration of the possible importance of fully understanding the natural history of the disease, including latent to declared disease, before accepting that screening is worthwhile. By the time a breast cancer reaches a size detectable by mammography, it has been estimated (assuming that a cancer starts in a single cell and that the doubling time of a cell in the body is similar to that observed in tissue cultures) that it may have been present for an average of nine years. It has also been estimated that only a further six months will elapse before it is detectable by touch. As what kills in breast cancer is metastasis, not the size of the original tumour, for screening to be efficacious one has to assume that in a substantial proportion of cases, the tumour has not metastasised for the first nine years of its existence, but will metastise at some point between being detectable by mammography and being detectable by touch. While this is possible, it is intrinsically unlikely and, without knowing the natural history of the disease, a screening programme is based on very uncertain foundations.

Agreeing whom should be treated as patients entails agreeing a definition of what constitutes a particular disease. For instance, at what level of blood pressure can someone be classed as 'hypertensive', ie having 'true' high blood pressure? And do the costs and benefits of a preventive programme make it a 'better buy' than other uses to which the staff, materials, buildings and money could be put? The benefits to patients of screening programmes are by no means self-evident and need to be carefully examined. For example, if there is no intervention of proven value for a particular disease, knowing that someone has that disease is probably irrelevant. And while some interventions may be worthwhile

111

in theory (efficacious) they may be poor in practice (ineffective). For instance, drugs with severe side-effects may not be taken as prescribed, or a diet may be so unpalatable that it is not adhered to. This is an important consideration which is often overlooked. There is, for example, pressure to introduce cholesterol screening for all adults, but there is no agreement among experts as to whether an effective treatment exists for those with moderately raised blood cholesterol levels.

The criteria for a screening programme are, on reflection, self-evident, but the fact that there are no fewer than 10 in all perhaps significantly reveals the gap between the common public perception of screening – that an attempt to catch a disease early must, by definition, be a good thing – and the more rigorous scientific requirement that screening programmes should work. Of course, some screening programmes will fulfil these criteria, and others will not and it is useful to examine a few instances in more detail.

Screening for PKU: an example of a programme which works well

PKU is a genetic defect of protein metabolism which occurs in 0.05–0.2 births per thousand. If untreated, serious permanent intellectual impairment results, placing an enormous strain on the individual, his or her carers and social and education services. Every individual in the UK is screened for PKU at birth, using a drop of blood obtained by a 'heel prick'. The drop is sent for a laboratory test highly specific to the disease and very sensitive to its presence. Individuals either have PKU or they do not. The test is easy and cheap and very acceptable; the population to be screened is available – almost 100 per cent of babies in the UK are delivered with the assistance of a health professional. A highly effective and cheap treatment is available: a diet which avoids certain foods. And, because parents are strongly motivated to avoid the very serious consequences of non-cooperation, the appropriate diet is followed. In other words, the programme for preventing the consequences of PKU works because it conforms well to all the criteria.

Screening for breast cancer – a programme that probably will not work

Now let us turn to breast cancer for which a national screening programme was set up just before the 1987 General Election. The contrasts in terms of the logistical problems in making this a success compared to that of PKU could not be more startling. First, women have to be invited for the test which requires a workable, computerised call/re-call scheme for which the take up rate is unlikely to be more than 60 per cent. The test or mammogram itself is acceptable to most women though it can be painful and has accordingly acquired the pejorative nickname of a 'boob squash'. The interpretation of the mammogram, however, requires a skilled radiographer and its specificity is poor – that is, perhaps one in a hundred abnormalities (perhaps more) considered to be suspicious, are in fact 'false positives' so there is need for them all to be biopsied. This is no easy task, as the 'tumours' are small and so difficult to locate, and requires skilled surgeons. Even the results of the biopsy are not necessarily clear-cut even to trained histopathologists which means that, erring on the side of caution, a proportion of those whose biopsies show equivocal evidence of breast cancer do not in fact have the disease. Finally, once the diagnosis is made, there is no consensus on the best way to treat it. Some surgeons recommend mastectomy, others lumpectomy and radio therapy, and others again would add-in cytotoxic drugs.

The cost of prevention programmes

Although 'prevention' is widely believed to be cheaper than 'cure' it can, in fact be considerably more expensive. For example, the cost of avoiding the birth of a child with spina bifida who would survive was estimated to be approximately £25,000 at 1984/85 prices, given the rate of disease which applies to most of England. And this example also illustrates other non-financial costs of screening programmes including the termination and loss of normal pregnancies as a consequence of false positives and as a side-effect of the second-stage investigation (amniocentesis) in the screening programme for spina bifida; and, more generally, inconvenience to patients and their families; the anxiety of patients and their families; and unnecessary treatment.

It is important not to concentrate on the unit cost of achieving the chosen outcome. It is a paradox of prevention programmes that they are cheap for each individual screened (eg, £10 for a cervical smear test) but expensive per outcome (eg, £300,000 per cervical cancer death avoided in Britain in the recent past). This is because most people being tested do not benefit from the test and the costs relating to the whole group have to be considered as 'transferred' to the person who benefits. In contrast, treatment programmes are expensive per individual but cheap per outcome because they are applied to relatively few people who are already known to have a problem. To be specific, let us compare the cost of two screening programmes – for PKU and cholesterol.

Screening for PKU by a heel-prick blood test can be done routinely at birth by a nurse without any specific training. The blood is routinely analysed, the result is unequivocal, the treatment of dietary restriction is highly efficacious. The 'costs' are thus those of the initial blood test, and subsequent ones if the baby is found to be affected; the cost of dietary advice and follow-up specialist consultations, and the not insubstantial social costs to child and parent of having to adhere to a strict dietary regime. The financial cost of ensuring a child with PKU does not suffer significant intellectual impairment works out at roughly £5,000.

The costs, by contrast, of a national cholesterol screening

programme include setting up some system to get the public to the surgery to have the blood test done. Then there are the costs of the blood test itself, which has to be repeated at regular intervals and, if 'abnormal', repeat tests to monitor treatment. There are the costs of the professional time of dieticians and doctors, and then the drug costs for those who fail to respond to dietary treatment.

To get some idea of what this costs in total, we can ignore the costs of the screening programme itself and just look at those of drug treatment. Taking the LRCCPPT trial of cholestyramine as an example, we find that the number of fatal heart attacks 'prevented' was eight, but the total cost of drug treatment for the duration of the trial was $8 million. This gives a figure of one million dollars for every life saved from heart disease. Unfortunately, no difference was observed in overall mortality between those who did and did not take the drug, which means the costs of saving a life may be infinite.

Conclusion

The sentiment which supports prevention uncritically is based on two fallacies:

- that prevention is better than cure;

- that prevention is cheaper than cure.

Examples have shown that both *can* be true (eg, screening for PKU) but often are not. Prevention is certainly not better than cure for normal foetuses aborted as a result of a spina bifida screening programme, or women having a cone biopsy of the cervix for lesions which will not progress to cancer, or people changing their lifestyle to one which does not suit them because they think they should. Each preventive programme must therefore be judged on its own individual merits and should neither be adopted nor ignored on grounds of sentiment.

A third fallacy plays a part in encouraging many people to

the view that prevention is so obviously desirable that to question it is eccentric and mischievous. This is the assumption that prevention is permanent avoidance of an event or (some of) its consequences, characteristically by a single act. When a road accident is 'prevented' by skilled driving it does not happen and we do not expect that an additional road accident will occur later as a consequence. But many 'prevention' programmes should really be called 'postponement' programmes. For example, coronary heart disease is, in general, delayed rather than avoided altogether; teeth that are well cared for eventually succumb to gum disease or decay, but do so later than they otherwise would. In 'postponement' programmes, not only is the event likely to happen in due course, but its continued postponement usually relies on continued action (such as continued adherence to a low-fat diet). Both of these factors increase costs, both non-monetary costs to the individual and monetary costs to society.

The complex chain of events in many prevention programmes has been illustrated. These chains are not even as strong as their weakest links; strength is the product of the weakness of all links. Suppose there is a 70 per cent chance a person will accept an invitation for screening, an 80 per cent chance that the test will find someone with a disease, a 50 per cent chance that the event which is the objective of the programme would otherwise occur in the person, a 75 per cent chance that it results in a change of lifestyle and a 50 per cent chance that such a change will delay the event, then the chances of the programme delaying the event are only 10.5 per cent ($.70 \times .80 \times .50 \times .75 \times .50$). 'Prevention chains' are typically much longer than 'treatment chains' and have to be effective for much longer periods of time. Prevention programmes are typically complex, requiring very good management and full cooperation by the patient. One must ask in each circumstance whether there are sufficient good managers and sufficient cooperative patients to make them work.

Recognising that the costs of prevention are non-monetary as well as monetary, and examining these costs is much better than creating programmes on the basis of an emotional pre-dilection for prevention as 'a good thing in itself'. By being more critical we can promote those that really work and avoid the harm caused by those that do not work, including the harm that wasted resources do to others who need services which cannot be funded as a result.

One of the difficulties is that we are trying to take decisions without adequate information. Most diseases are, in fact, rare, even if they are thought to be common. It has been calculated that a study to decide whether screening for cervical cancer should be carried out at one-year rather than five-year inter-vals, would require almost one million women, because cervi-cal cancer does not occur often in a population and because there is likely to be only a small difference in the two pro-cedures – if any at all.

It is not always better to make a diagnosis earlier rather than later. If treating someone earlier in the course of the disease does not improve the length or quality of life, discovering the disease through a screening test is of no benefit and may actually be counter-productive if it causes unnecessary anxiety.

The Ethics of Prevention

Petr Skrabanek

Medical ethics

What is the ethical basis for the idea, now universally accepted, that those who smoke and drink and take no exercise are morally inferior to those who watch their weight, drink fizzy water and go to the gym three times a week?

Jane Ellison

The physician is not the servant of science or of the race, or even of life. He is the individual servant of his individual patients, basing his decisions always on their individual interest.

Theodore Fox

The behaviour of doctors was, and largely is, governed by professional etiquette: not sleeping with patients, not splitting fees, not advertising, not operating when drunk. Awareness of ethical principles and constraints is very recent. Guidelines on informed consent and on experimentation with humans have only appeared in the past few decades as a response to public pressure following a series of medical scandals.

Medical ethics is founded on four pillars: non-maleficence, beneficence, autonomy and justice. The principle of non-maleficence, that is, of not doing harm to patients, dates back to the Hippocratic-Galenic *primum non nocere* (at least do no harm), though what this precept actually meant is far from clear.[1] The positive corollary to non-maleficence is beneficence, that is, of acting only in the interest of the patient. This principle is under threat when a doctor serves two masters, the patient and the state.[2] When the common good takes precedence over individual good, people are turned into statistical numbers, to be manipulated in the name of the nation's bright future. Breaches of the principle of beneficence can be daily encountered, for example when patients serve as a means for completing a 'project', for the advancement of one's career, or for increasing one's income. Medicine, and that includes health promotion, in Western countries is becoming increasingly profit-driven and self-serving.

The principle of autonomy implies an unfettered right to make decisions about one's own life, even if such decisions are seen by others as 'foolish'. Doctors' beneficence without patient autonomy is paternalism. As John Stuart Mill noted, paternalism is justified in the case of real parents, since they have affection for their children and, presumably, superiority in wisdom and experience. But what doctor, acting in the interest of the nation's health, has affection for those waiting to be screened? What doctor has more wisdom and experience when it comes to the art of living? Do doctors have happier marriages, more peaceful minds, more blissful deaths? The danger of paternalism lies not so much in its abuse of unmandated power, as in the insidiousness of making people happier and healthier against their will.

The final principle, that of justice, governs the equal right of everyone to medical care, regardless of whether their disease is 'deserved' or whether they are 'innocent victims'. To claim, however, that everyone has a 'fundamental right' to complete physical, mental and social well-being, as the WHO proclaims, is a nonsense upon stilts. In the context of health promotion, distributive justice demands that limited health resources are not wasted on activities of little or no benefit, when time and money could be spent more effectively on caring for the queues of the sick.

PREVENTIONITIS

Should prevention carry a health warning?

They that are whole need not a physician.
St Matthew (ix, 12)

Prevention *may* be better than cure, provided that the benefits outweigh the harm. In an ethical context the harm may result from loss of autonomy, from maleficence (when the preventive measure does more harm than good), and from maldistribution of medical resources, when too high a cost is paid for a meagre result. A pound of prevention is not worth a penn'orth of cure.

One of the reasons why prevention has become so popular among politicians is a mistaken belief that in time it would reduce the health budget. Even in the case of smoking, where a reduction in tobacco consumption would prevent some premature deaths, 'the economic benefits of tobacco far outweigh the health care costs'.[3] Premature death from lung cancer is less expensive than continuing pensions and the protracted death of institutionalised senescence.

According to the new General Practitioner contract, doctors are required to establish health promotion clinics and carry out health checks, within 28 days, in all new patients or in patients who have not had a health check in the last 12 months. The cost-effectiveness of such activities has never been assessed and is thus unknown,[4] but in the only British randomised controlled trial of regular health checks in middle-aged people, the group allotted to health screening had slightly higher mortality from cancer, cardiovascular disease and all causes combined, than the unscreened control group. The authors concluded that

> since these control trial results have failed to demonstrate any beneficial effect on either mortality or morbidity, we believe that the use of general-practice based multiphasic

screening in the middle-aged can no longer be advocated on scientific, ethical or economic grounds as a desirable public health measure.[5]

Preventionists put the common good before the individual good, using a crude utilitarian calculus. Since their assumptions of benefit are often insupportable or wrong, imaginary numbers of 'lives saved' are conjured from their magician's hat. One of the leading British epidemiologists calculated that if the British people used less salt, 70,000 lives would be saved annually.[6]

Benefits to statistical persons must be set against harms inflicted upon people with a name and an address. Geoffrey Rose introduced the notion of the so-called 'prevention paradox', according to which 'a measure that brings large benefits to the community offers little to each participating individual'.[7] This formulation is misleading, as it suggests that the benefit is equally distributed. In fact, a small number of individuals, if the benefit were real, would gain from prevention, while the large majority would not benefit at all, though all of them would run the risk of being harmed. Frederic Bastiat, the 19th century political thinker, made a similar observation with regard to trade protection: 'Protection concentrates at a single point the good that it does, while the harm that it inflicts is diffused over a wide area'.[8] Thus, to use an illustrative example, if a person is found on screening to have a risk factor which, based on statistical averages, would confer on him a one in 10 probability of developing the disease during his lifetime, and an early intervention is being offered which would reduce this risk by 50 per cent, then out of 100 persons with such a risk factor, 90 would never incur the disease and 95 would be treated without any benefit. But once 'at risk', always at risk, and all 100 would have to live with such a label, which by means of spurious reification, becomes part of the person, a 'ticking-bomb within', so to speak. In the case of coronary heart disease, some 300 risk factors have been described, yet randomised controlled trials in which the simultaneous modification of the major risk factors was attempted, failed to show any benefits to the subjects of these experiments.[9]

In a further bizarre twist, preventionists now argue that even people with normal weight, normal blood pressure, or an average alcohol consumption should try to do one step better, so that the population mean for these 'risk factors' would be lowered. To use their own words, 'it is no longer possible to regard *normal* behaviour as of no wider consequence'.[10] The whole nation is to become a patient, for whom a 'national diet' is to be prescribed, so that the 'national cholesterol' is right. On an even larger scale, similar plans are being drawn up for the whole of Europe and ultimately for the whole world by the WHO.[11] It was Henri de Mondeville, a 13th century French surgeon, who observed that anyone who believes that the same thing can be suited to everyone is a great fool, since medicine is practised not on mankind in general but on every individual in particular.

It is not widely appreciated that 'preventive' measures can prove disastrous. For example, in 1976 President Ford asked Congress to earmark $135 million towards to cost of swine-flu vaccine, to inoculate 'every man, woman and child in the United States'. In the end, some 50 million Americans received the vaccine before the programme came to a sudden halt because of the appearance of serious neurological complications in more than 500 people, of whom 32 died. The net cost to the taxpayer was in the region of one billion dollars, and the government faced compensation claims for three billion dollars. The whole swine-flu fiasco had all the hallmarks of zealous prevention untempered with prudence. The scare was based on a single outbreak among military recruits, one of whom died on a night march. No critics were invited to the 'consensus' conferences at which the 'blueprint for action' was drafted. It was an election year, and President Ford wished to be seen as someone who cared deeply for people's health. The vaccine was administered without clear, informed consent, and possible side-effects of an untested vaccine were played down by public health officials.[12]

In the case of vaccination, at least the nature of infection is understood. When it comes to chronic degenerative diseases, such as coronary heart disease or cancer, the aetiology of which is not understood, blunderbuss intervention in 'life-style', or attempts to modify 'risk factors' are likely to fail. Yet medical interventions to prevent coronary heart disease or cancer are accepted automatically as beneficial or, at least, as not doing any harm. There are, however, many examples which gainsay this cosy belief.

Hundreds of thousands of people received the drug tri-paranol in the hope of preventing heart disease, with the reported net result that about 1,000 of them developed cataract and many more became impotent.[13] The drug clofibrate, believed to prevent heart disease by reducing blood cholesterol, was given to 5,000 men on a long-term basis; to the surprise of the investigators, significantly more men died who were allocated to clofibrate than among the controls.[14] In a more recent example from Finland, 1,200 healthy business executives were randomised into a control group or a multiple-risk-factor intervention group, in an attempt to prove that such an intervention prevents coronary heart disease. In fact, significantly more men in the intervention group died of coronary heart disease than in the control group.[15]

Prevention enthusiasts take no notice of experimental re-futations of their belief that prevention is 'good'. In many countries, community-based programmes of intervention are instituted, without any possibility of evaluating them and without informing the participants that the programme is not for their own good. Non-participation ('non-compliance' in the paternalistic jargon) implies irresponsibility.

When population screening programmes are introduced, usually with the intention of screening the sexual organs of women, it is assumed that every woman should be responsible enough to avail herself of such a programme. Yet how many women are informed by the screeners of the accuracy of the offered test? In a letter to *The Times* (3 December, 1992) a group of MPs complained that 'every year between 500,000 and 750,000 women are misled by their smear test result'. How many people realise that a test which is 98 per cent specific and 100 per cent sensitive (that is, it correctly identifies all the people with the disease, and gives two false-positive results among 1,000 people who do not have the disease), when applied to a population with a prevalence of the tested disease of one in 1,000 (such as more common cancers), is wrong in 95 out 100 positive tests and that the Pap smear is even less accurate?[16]

The ethical vacuum of preventive medicine

The preventive function of government, however, is far more liable to be abused, to the prejudice of liberty, than the punitive function; for there is hardly any part of the legitimate freedom of action of a human being which would not admit of being represented, and fairly, too, as increasing the facilities for some form or other of delinquency.

John Stuart Mill

As the scope of 'prevention' now extends far beyond strictly medical conditions, and intrudes into the area of human behaviour and beliefs, it is surprising that professional ethicists have not devoted at least part of their intellectual effort to devise safeguards which would protect whole populations from unwarranted experiments, conducted by governments or their agents in the name of 'health promotion', as defined by the WHO, that is, encompassing their physical, mental, social (and spiritual?) well-being.

Some headway has been made in restricting experimentation with human volunteers, mainly due to many public scandals which publicised the use of humans as 'guinea pigs', such as the Tuskegee study, conducted by the US Public Health Service for 40 years on blacks with syphilis, who were denied treatment,[17] the secret experiments in which thousands of soldiers and civilians where unwittingly exposed to LSD,[18] the exposure of patients to radioactive materials without their consent,[19] and many others.[20]

Paradoxically, the strict guidelines governing experimentation on human volunteers or patients have never been extended to experimentation on whole populations, even though the potential harm could be much greater because of the much larger numbers involved. An apparent reason for this discrepancy must be the widely accepted notion that if it is 'prevention' it must be good, and therefore the usual ethical constraints do not apply. As mentioned above, whether prevention is 'good' or not, begs the question, and requires a rigorous proof in each particular instance.

Doubts about the notion that many preventive measures are in fact experimental in nature can be dissipated by pointing out that it is deemed ethical to assess their efficacy in randomised controlled trials. How might this work in practice? It is now an essential principle of ethical medicine that patients be informed of the pros and cons of medical treatment or, if surgery is proposed, that their consent be obtained. There seems no good reason why the same principle should not hold for preventive measures like mass media campaigns and screening programmes.

Mass media campaigns should be obliged to reflect the scientific claims on which they are based. Campaigns promoting a healthy diet as a means of preventing coronary heart disease would have to point out that 'the effectiveness of this advice has not been confirmed by medical trials'. Furthermore, even if a preventive programme is shown to be beneficial, it still is not a sufficient reason for its introduction without informed consent of the potential participants.

As for screening programmes, in the US, with its hypertrophied legal profession, it is now envisaged that physicians who fail to disclose the pros and cons of a suggested procedure may be sued for 'dignitary tort', that is, for affronting the patient's dignity by preventing him or her from exercising his or her right to rational participation.[21]

More recently, in Britain, a lawyer and a paediatrician have suggested that

> failure to obtain informed consent for a screening procedure is not only ethically unacceptable but also exposes the health authority to the risk of litigation [and that] failure to provide adequate information for the subject to give informed consent may not only result in an action for negligence but also lead to an action for trespass against the person.[22]

In an accompanying editorial comment, the editor emphasised that 'those who propose changes in whole populations must be even more sure of their ground than those who seek changes in individual people'.

It would seem essential that in breast and cervical screening programmes, the doctors' responsibility should be not only to seek their patients' permission, but also their consent, which should be voluntary, competent, informed and understanding. As informed consent is meant primarily to protect the doctor (the patient does not even receive a copy), a further protection of the participant in any preventive screening or other preventive measure, could be provided by a written form, signed by the doctor, describing the accuracy of the test, the probability of benefit and the probability and the nature of adverse outcomes.

As it is unlikely that the health promotion industry will get its house in order without outside pressure, a forum should be set up, at which representatives of the public and of the medical and legal professions would identify the ethical problems of prevention and draw up guidelines for protecting the public against unethical practices.[23]

Notes and references

Chapter 2
1. W G Guntheroth, *JAMA*, 1992, 267, 235.
2. Department of Health, *Health of the Nation*, HMSO, 1992.
3. P Tsais et al, *American Journal of Public Health*, 1978, 68, 966.
4. E Jannerfeltte, *British Medical Journal*, 1988, 296, 278.
5. A Bradford Hill, *A Short Textbook of Medical Statistics*, London 1977.
6. R Doll and R Peto, *The Causes of Cancer*, Oxford University Press, 1981.
7. V A Study, *JAMA*, 1967, 202, 116.
8. G Davey Smith, *British Medical Journal*, 1993, 306, 1367.

Chapter 4
1. Department of Health, *Health of the Nation*, HMSO, 1992.
2. Ibid, p 34.
3. Roy Griffiths, *Management Inquiry*, 1983.
4. Ibid, p 33.
5. Department of Health, op cit.
6. Secretary of State for Health *Working for Patients*, Command 555, London: HMSO, 1989.

Chapter 6
1. Consensus Conference, 'Lowering blood cholesterol to prevent heart disease', *JAMA*, 1985, 253, 2080–2086.
2. British Cardiac Society Working Group on Coronary Prevention, 'Conclusions and recommendations', *British Heart Journal*, 1987, 57, 188–189.
3. Study Group, European Atherosclerosis Society, 'Strategies for the prevention of coronary heart disease: a policy statement of the European Atherosclerosis Society', *European Heart Journal*, 1987, 8, 77–88.
4. J Shepherd, D J Betteridge, P Durrington, et al, 'Strategies for reducing coronary heart disease and desirable limits for blood lipid

concentrations: guidelines of the British Hyperlipidaemia Association', *British Medical Journal*, 1987, 295, 1245–1246.

5. The Expert Panel, 'Report of the National Cholesterol Education Programme Expert Panel on detection, evaluation and treatment of high blood cholesterol in adults', *Archives of Internal Medicine*, 1988, 148, 36–39.

6. Standing Medical Advisory Committee, *Blood cholesterol testing. The cost effectiveness of opportunistic cholesterol testing*, Department of Health, 1990.

7. Royal College of General Practitioners Working Party, 'Guidelines for the Management of Hyperlipidaemia in General Practice. Towards the Primary Prevention of Coronary Heart Disease', *Occasional Paper 55*, Royal College of General Practitioners, London, 1992.

8. H A Tyroler, 'Overview of clinical trials of cholesterol lowering in relationship to epidemiologic studies', *American Journal of Medicine*, 1988, 87, Supplement 4A, 14S–19S.

9. Refs 1–7 op cit.

10. L E Ramsay, W W Yeo and P R Jackson, 'Dietary reduction of serum cholesterol: time to think again', *British Medical Journal*, 1991, 303, 953–957.

11. Ibid.

12. Multiple Risk Factor Intervention Trial Research Group, 'Multiple Risk Factor Intervention Trial. Risk factor changes and mortality results', *JAMA*, 1982, 248, 1465–1477.

13. Ramsay, Yeo and Jackson, op cit.

14. Royal College of General Practitioners Working Party op cit.

15. U Ravnskov, 'Cholesterol lowering trials in coronary heart disease: frequency of citation and outcome', *British Medical Journal*, 1992, 305, 15–19.

16. J G Schmidt, 'Cholesterol lowering treatment and mortality', *British Medical Journal*, 1992, 305, 1226–1227.

17. M F Muldoon, S B Manuck and K A Matthews, 'Lowering cholesterol concentrations and mortality: a quantitative review of primary prevention trials', *British Medical Journal*, 1990, 301, 309–314.

18. A G Shaper, S J Pocock, A N Phillips and M Walker, 'Identifying men at risk of heart attacks: strategy for use in general practice', *British Medical Journal*, 1986, 293, 474–479.

19. I Robertson, A Phillips, D Mant et al, 'Motivational effect of cholesterol measurement in general practice health checks', *British Journal of General Practice*, 1992, 42, 469–472.

20. S B Hulley, J M B Walsh and T B Newman, 'Health Policy on Blood Cholesterol. Time to Change Directions', *Circulation*, 1992, 86, 1026–1029.

21. Committee of Principal Investigators, 'A cooperative trial of primary

prevention of ischaemic heart disease using clofibrate', *British Heart Journal*, 1978, 40, 1069–1118.

Chapter 7
1. Department of Health, *Health of the Nation*, HMSO, 1992.
2. J Newton and T K H Craig, 'Prevention', in D H Bennett and H L Freeman (eds), *Community Psychiatry*, Edinburgh: Churchill Livingstone, 1991.
3. R F Mollica, 'Community mental health centres. An American response to Kathleen Jones', *Journal of the Royal Society of Medicine*, 1980, 73, 863–870.
4. J E Cooper, 'Crisis admission units and emergency psychiatric services', *Public Health in Europe II*, Copenhagen: World Health Organization Regional Office for Europe, 1979.
5. J Leff, 'Principles of Social Psychiatry', in D Bhugra and J Leff (eds), *Principle of Social Psychiatry*, Oxford: Blackwell, 1993.
6. Newton and Craig, op cit.
7. T S Bhugra, 'Social Support Networks', in Bhugra and Leff, op cit.
8. Department of Health, op cit.
9. National Institute for Mental Health, *Towards a Model for a Comprehensive Community-based Mental Health System*, Washington DC: NIMH, 1987.
10. F Holloway, 'Caring for People, a critical review of British Government policy for the mentally ill', *Psychiatric Bulletin*, 14, 641–645, 1990.
11. M W Linn, E M Caffey, J Klett, G E Hogarty and H R Lamb, 'Day treatment and psychotropic drugs in the aftercare of scizophrenic patients', *Archives of General Psychiatry*, 1979, 36, 1055–1066.
12. L I Stein and M A Test, 'Alternative to mental hospital treatment', *Archives of General Psychiatry*, 1980, 37, 392–397; M Muijen, I M Marks, J Connelly, B Audini and G McNamee, 'The Daily Living Programme. Preliminary comparison of community versus hospital-based treatment for the seriously mentally ill facing emergency admission', *British Journal of Psychiatry*, 1992, 160, 379–384; F Creed, D Black, P Anthony, M Osborn, P Thomas and B Tomenson, 'Randomised controlled trial of day patient versus inpatient psychiatric treatment', *British Medical Journal*, 1990, 300, 1033–1037.
13. F Holloway, A M Silverman and A W Wainwright, 'Not Waving but Drowning. The East Lambeth Inpatient Survey 1990', *International Journal of Social Psychiatry*, 1992, 38, 131–137.
14. Holloway, 1990, op cit.
15. L Davidson and J S Strauss, 'Sense of self in recovery from severe mental illness', *British Journal of Medical Psychology*, 1992, 65, 131–145.

16. J Kanter, 'The process of change in the long-term mentally ill: a naturalistic perspective', *Psychosocial Rehabilitation Journal*, 1985, 9, 55–69.
17. Social Services Inspectorate, *Care Management and Assessment. Manager's Guide*, London: HMSO, 1991.
18. S Nicholson, 'Suicide in North Devon: epidemic or problem of classification?', *Health Trends*, 1992, 24, 95–96.
19. K Michel and L Valach, 'Suicide prevention: spreading the gospel to General Practitioners', *British Journal of Psychiatry*, 1992, 160, 757–760.
20. H G Morgan and P Priest, 'Suicide and other unexpected deaths among psychiatric inpatients. The Bristol Confidential Inquiry', *British Journal of Psychiatry*, 1991, 158, 368–374.
21. M Patrick, A Higgit, F Holloway and M Silverman, 'Changes in an Inner City Psychiatric Inpatient Service Following Bed Losses: a follow-up of the East Lambeth 1986 Survey', *Health Trends*, 1989, 21, 121–123.

Chapter 8
1. L W Green, *Health Education Monograph*, 1970, no. 30.
2. J A Jaccard, *Health Education Monograph*, 1975, 3:2.
3. H Leventhal, *American Cardiology*, 1973, 31, 571.
4. A Gatherer et al, *Is Health Education Effective?*, HEC, 1978.
5. R Patterson et al, *The Lancet*, 1958, 2, 791.
6. Research Survey of GB Ltd, *Tar and Nicotine HEC advertising campaigns 1974, 1975, 1976* (Mimeo).
7. *Adult Use of Tobacco*, Report for the Bureau of Health Education Department, HEW, USA, 1975.
8. Communication Research Ltd, *A Study of the Effects of the HEC 1974 anti-alcohol campaign in Tyne-Tees* (Mimeo).
9. C Winnick, *General Psychology*, 1973, 68, 289.
10. J Bond, *Smoking in Pregnancy*, Report from Strathclyde Area Survey, 1977 (Mimeo).
11. M Plant, *Journal of Social Psychology*, 1978.
12. Research Services Ltd, *Anti-smoking advertising report: Report of HEC Anti-smoking campaign 1972* (Mimeo).
13. J G Richards, *Public Education about Cancer*, UICC, 1977.
14. Kolskeke et al, *International Journal of Health Education* 1976, 19, 59.
15. J W Farquhar, *The Lancet*, 1977, 1, 119–122.
16. K Warner, *Journal of Public Health*, 1977, 67, 645.
17. National Advisory Committee on Nutrition Education, *Report*, London, 1983.
18. World Health Organization, *Statistics Annual*, Geneva: WHO, 1952–1984.

19. Mr Fit Research Group, *JAMA*, 1982, 248, 1465.
20. Food and Agriculture Organization, *Year Book*, Rome: FAO, 1982.
21. M Terris, *American Journal of Public Health*, 1967, 57, 207.
22. R Golupjatnikov et al, *The Lancet*, 1983, 2, 681.
23. V C Riley, *The Lancet*, 1991, 337, 183.
24. CTR Report, 1993, 3, 77.
25. N Ford, *British Journal of Family Planning*, 1993, 18, 119.

Chapter 10

1. A R Jones, 'Do no harm', *Annals of Internal Medicine*, 1978, 88, 827–832.
2. P Skrabanek, 'The physician's responsibility to the patient', *The Lancet*, 1988, 1, 1155–1157.
3. P Taylor, *The smoke ring*, London: Sphere Books, 1985.
4. T Scott and A Maynard, *Will the new GP contract lead to cost-effective medical practice?*, Discussion paper 83, University of York: Centre for Health Economics, 1991.
5. W W Holland, A L Creese, M F D'Souza, et al, 'A controlled trial of multiphasic screening in middle-age: results of the South-East London screening study', *International Journal of Epidemiology*, 1977, 6, 357–363.
6. M R Law, C D Frost and N J Wald, 'Analysis of data from trials on salt reduction', *British Medical Journal*, 1991, 302, 819–824.
7. G Rose, 'Strategy of prevention: lessons from cardiovascular disease', *British Medical Journal*, 1981, 282, 1847–1851.
8. F Bastiat, quoted in T S Szasz, *Our right to drugs: the case for a free market*, New York: Praeger, 1992.
9. J McCormick and P Skrabanek, 'Coronary heart disease is not preventable by population interventions', *The Lancet*, 1988, 2, 839–841.
10. G Rose and S Day, 'The population mean predicts the number of deviant individuals', *British Medical Journal*, 1990, 301, 1031–1034.
11. P Skrabanek, 'Dietary guidelines: WHO makes them; who reads them? Who needs them?' in *Who Needs WHO? Three views on the World Health Organization's dietary guidelines*, London: Social Affairs Unit, 1992, 7–20.
12. D B Dutton, *Worse than the disease. Pitfalls of medical progress*, Cambridge: Cambridge University Press, 1988.
13. E C Lambert, *Modern medical mistakes*, Bloomington: Indiana University Press, 1978.
14. Committee of Principal Investigators, 'WHO cooperative trial on primary prevention of ischaemic heart disease using clofibrate to lower serum cholesterol: mortality follow-up', *The Lancet*, 1980, 2, 379–385.
15. T E Strandberg, V V Salomaa, V A Naukkarinen, H T Vanbannen, S J Sarna and T A Miettinen, 'Long-term mortality after 5-year multi-

factorial primary prevention of cardiovascular diseases in middle-aged men', *JAMA* 1991, 266, 1225–1229.

16. P Skrabanek, 'Cervical cytology screening: the case against', *Advances in Obstetrics and Gynaecology*, 1991, 3, 17–21.
17. J H Jones, *Bad blood. The Tuskegee syphilis experiment*, New York: Free Press, 1981.
18. G J Annas, *The rights of patients*, New York: American Civil Liberties Union, 1992.
19. US House of Representatives Sub-committee, *American nuclear guinea pigs: three decades of radiation experiments on US citizens*, Washington DC: US Government Printing Office, 1986.
20. H K Beecher, 'Ethics and clinical research', *New England Journal of Medicine*, 1966, 274, 1354–1360; M H Pappworth, *Human guinea pigs. Experimentation on man*, Harmondsworth: Penguin Books, 1969.
21. G J Annas, op cit.
22. P J Edwards and D M Hall, 'Screening, ethics and the law', *British Medical Journal*, 1992, 305, 267–268.
23. R Gillon, 'Ethics in health promotion and prevention of disease', *Journal of Medical Ethics*, 1990, 16, 171–172; P Skrabanek, 'Why is preventive medicine exempted from ethical constraints?' *Journal of Medical Ethics*, 1990, 16, 187–190.

THE SOCIAL AFFAIRS UNIT

The SAU is a research and educational trust committed to the promotion of lively and wide-ranging debate on social affairs. Its authors – now numbering over 150 – have analysed the factors which make for a free and orderly society in which enterprise can flourish. Over the last two years it has been increasingly involved in joint UK/US ventures, including *Health, Lifestyle and Environment: Countering the Panic* with the Manhattan Institute, and *The Loss of Virtue: Moral Confusion and Social Disorder in Britain and America*, now published as a **National Review** book. Current areas of work include consumer affairs, the critical appraisal of welfare and public spending and problems of freedom and personal responsibility.

The Unit's impact and funding

The Times writes:

> *The Social Affairs Unit is famous for driving its coach and horses through the liberal consensus, scattering intellectual picket lines as it goes. It is equally famous for raising questions which strike most people most of the time as too dangerous or too difficult to think about.*

To maintain its independence, the Unit is funded by a wide range of foundations and trusts, sales of its publications and corporate donations from highly diverse sectors. It has received support from some 80 sources. The SAU is registered as an educational charity, number 281530.

SOME PUBLICATIONS FROM
THE SOCIAL AFFAIRS UNIT

On education . . .

Educational Achievement in Japan: Lessons for The West
Richard Lynn
'. . . finds that teacher motivation
in Japan is fuelled by two factors:
having to teach to a national
curriculum and working in schools
which have to compete on results
to survive.'
　　Times Educational Supplement
STUDIES IN SOCIAL REVALUATION 1
*Published in cooperation with
The Macmillan Press*
Casebound:
ISBN 0 333 44531 7　£29.50
Paperback:
ISBN 0 333 44532 5　£8.95

The Wayward Curriculum: A cause for parents' concern?
Edited by Dennis O'Keeffe
'This excellent collection'
　　　*Times Higher Education
　　　　　　　　Supplement*
ISBN 0 907631 19 3
£9.95 casebound

Schooling for British Muslims: Integrated, opted-out or denominational?
Mervyn Hiskett
'A reasoned case in favour of
creating separate state-funded
Muslim schools'
　　　　　　　　The Times
RESEARCH REPORT 12
ISBN 0 907631 33 9　£4.50

Trespassing? Businessmen's views on the education system
Michael Brophy et al
ISBN 0 907631 11 8　£2.95

Educated for Employment?
Digby Anderson et al
ISBN 0 907631 03 7　£2.65

The Pied Pipers of Education
Antony Flew et al
ISBN 0 907631 02 9　£2.65

Who Teaches the Teachers? A contribution to public debate of the DES Green Paper
Anthony O'Hear
RESEARCH REPORT 10
ISBN 0 907631 31 2　£3.00

Detecting Bad Schools: a guide for normal parents
Digby Anderson
ISBN 0 907631 04 5　£1.00

On Law and order . . .

Deterring Potential Criminals
Ernest van den Haag
'Will most probably have a
considerable influence'
　　　*Howard Journal of Criminal
　　　　　　　　　　Justice*
RESEARCH REPORT 7
ISBN 0 907361 14 2　£2.00

Criminal Welfare on Trial
Colin Brewer et al
ISBN 0 907631 01 1　£2.65

Are the Police Under Control?
David Regan
RESEARCH REPORT 1
ISBN 0 907631 06 1　£1.00

Are the Police Fair?
P A J Waddington
RESEARCH REPORT 2
ISBN 907631 07 X £1.00

On the Welfare State . . .

A Phantom Carnage: the myth that low income kills
James Le Fanu
RESEARCH REPORT 17
ISBN 0 907631 51 7 £5.00

Magic in the Surgery Counselling in the NHS: a licensed state friendship service
Myles Harris
RESEARCH REPORT 20
ISBN 0 907631 56 8 £5.00

Popular Attitudes to State Welfare Services: a growing demand for alternatives?
Peter Saunders and Colin Harris
'suggest[s] that the public feels "trapped" into supporting state services by taxation because people are unable or unwilling to pay twice'   *Sunday Times*
RESEARCH REPORT 11
ISBN 0 907631 30 4 £3.00

Action on Welfare: reform of personal income taxation and social security
Hermione Parker
RESEARCH REPORT 4
ISBN 0 907361 04 5 £2.00

Breaking The Spell Of The Welfare State
Digby Anderson, June Lait & David Marsland
ISBN 0 907631 00 2 £2.65

On family matters . . .

Families in Dreamland: Challenging the new consensus for state childcare
Patricia Morgan
RESEARCH REPORT 15
ISBN 0 907631 48 7 £4.00

Full Circle? Bringing up children in the post-permissive society
Edited by Digby Anderson
ISBN 0 907631 29 0 £8.95

Denying Homes to Black Children: Britain's new race adoption policies
David Dale
RESEARCH REPORT 8
ISBN 0 907631 32 1 £3.50

On risk and health . . .

Environmental Alarums: a medical audit of environmental damage to human health
James Le Fanu
RISK CONTROVERSIES 3
ISBN 0 907631 57 6 £5.00

Risk Health and the Consumer
James McCormick and Digby Anderson
RISK CONTROVERSIES 1
ISBN 0 907631 47 9 £3.50

Health, Lifestyle and Environment: Countering the Panic
Produced in cooperation with the Manhattan Institute
'suggests that the nation is gripped by a "health panic" generated by often contradictory advice from researchers'
                    The Times
ISBN 0 907631 44 4 £9.95

A Diet of Reason: sense and nonsense in the healthy eating debate
Edited by Digby Anderson
Casebound:
ISBN 0 907631 26 6   £9.95
Paperback:
ISBN 0 907631 22 3   £5.95

Drinking to Your Health: the allegations and the evidence
Edited by Digby Anderson
Casebound:
ISBN 0 007631 37 1   £14.95
Paperback:
ISBN 0 907631 38 X   £9.95

On international organizations . . .

Chattering International: how Unicef fails the world's poorest children
James Le Fanu
RESEARCH REPORT 19
ISBN 0 907631 53 3   £5.00

Who Benefits from WHO: the decline of the World Health Organization
Robert D Tollison and Richard E Wagner
RESEARCH REPORT 18
ISBN 0 907631 55 X   £5.00

Who needs WHO? Three views on the World Health Organization's Dietary Guidelines
Petr Skrabanek et al
RESEARCH REPORT 16
ISBN 0 907631 49 5   £5.00

On the environment and housing . . .

After Government Failure?
D R Denman
TAKING THOUGHT FOR THE ENVIRONMENT 1
ISBN 0 907631 24 X   £2.50

Planning Fails the Inner Cities
R N Goodchild and D R Denman
TAKING THOUGHT FOR THE ENVIRONMENT 2
ISBN 0 907631 25 8   £2.50

Caring for the Countryside: public dependence on private interest
Barry Bracewell-Milnes
TAKING THOUGHT FOR THE ENVIRONMENT 3
ISBN 0 907631 27 4   £2.50

Home Truths
Barbara Robson et al
ISBN 0 907631 05 3   £2.95

Asian Housing in Britain
Jon Davies
RESEARCH REPORT 6
ISBN 0 907631 13 4   £2.00

On moral and social issues . . .

The Loss of Virtue: Moral confusion and social disorder in Britain and America
Edited by Digby Anderson
A NATIONAL REVIEW BOOK
ISBN 0 907631 50 9   £15.95

Finding Fault in Divorce
George Brown
MORAL ASPECTS OF SOCIAL PROBLEMS 1
ISBN 0 907631 32 0   £3.50

Why Social Policy Cannot be Morally Neutral: the current confusion about pluralism
Basil Mitchell
MORAL ASPECTS OF SOCIAL PROBLEMS 2
ISBN 0 907631 35 5   £3.50

Self-Improvement and Social Action
Antony Flew
MORAL ASPECTS OF SOCIAL PROBLEMS 3
ISBN 0 907631 36 3   £3.50

Consumer Debt: whose responsibility?
K Alec Chrystal
MORAL ASPECTS OF SOCIAL PROBLEMS 4
ISBN 0 907631 39 8   £3.50

Do Animals Have Rights?
Tibor Machan
MORAL ASPECTS OF SOCIAL PROBLEMS 5
ISBN 0 907631 40 1   £3.50

The Unmentionable Face of Poverty in the Nineties: domestic incompetence, improvidence and male irresponsibility in low income families
Digby Anderson
THE MORAL DIMENSION OF SOCIAL POLICY
ISBN 0 907631 42 8   £4.00

The Kindness that Kills: the churches' simplistic response to complex social issues
Edited by Digby Andreson
Commissioned by the SAU and published by SPCK
ISBN 0 281 04096 6   £3.95

Wealth And Poverty: a Jewish analysis
Jonathan Sacks
TAKING THOUGHT FOR THE POOR 1
ISBN 0 907631 15 0   £2.00

The Bible, Justice and the Culture of Poverty: emotive calls to action versus rational analysis
Irving Hexham
TAKING THOUGHT FOR THE POOR 2
ISBN 0 907631 16 9   £2.00

The Philosophy of Poverty: Good Samaritans or Procrusteans?
Antony Flew
TAKING THOUGHT FOR THE POOR 3
ISBN 0 907631 17 7   £2.00

The Christian Response To Poverty: working with God's economic laws
James Sadowsky
TAKING THOUGHT FOR THE POOR 4
ISBN 0 907631 18 5   £2.00

On economic matters . . .

The Secret of the Miracle Economy: different national attitudes to competitiveness and money
Richard Lynn
'reports only "competitiveness" is significantly connected with economic growth' *Financial Times*
ISBN 0 907631 41 X   £8.95

Set Fair: a gradualist proposal for privatising weather forecasting
Jerome Ellig
RESEARCH REPORT 13
ISBN 0 907631 34 7   £4.50

On the media and advertising . . .

**Reaching for the Counter
The new child consumers:
regulation or education?**
Adrian Furnham
RISK CONTROVERSIES 2
ISBN 0 907631 54 1   £7.50

**Advertising Bans: administrative
decisions or matters of principle**
John Gray
ISBN 0 907631 43 6   £4.00

**Advertising Bans: consequences for
consumers**
Mark Bentley and Mai Fyfield
ISBN 0 907631 45 2   £4.00

**The Megaphone Solution:
government attempts to cure social
problems with mass media
campaigns**
Digby Anderson
'will undoubtedly cause a furore'
                                        Marketing
RESEARCH REPORT 9
ISBN 0 907631 28 2   £3.00

**Tracts Beyond The Times: a brief
guide to the communist or
revolutionary Marxist press**
Charles Ellwell
RESEARCH REPORT 3
ISBN 0 907631 08 8   £1.50

On affirmative action . . .

A Future for Anti-Racism?
Antony Flew
RESEARCH REPORT 14
ISBN 0 90763 46 0   £4.00

**Reversing Racism: lessons from
America**
*Kenneth M Holland & Geoffrey
Parkins*
RESEARCH REPORT 5
ISBN 0 907631 10 X   £2.00

And . . .

Extra Dry: columns in The Times
Digby Anderson
'imperative writing on political
and social subjects.' *The Spectator*
ISBN 0 907631 12 6   £2.95